GREEN MAGIC
The Healing Power
of
Herbs, Talismans, and Stones

Other books by Morwyn:

Secrets of a Witch's Coven
Web of Light: Rites for Witches in the New Age

Morwyn

GREEN MAGIC
The Healing Power
of
Herbs, Talismans, and Stones

MORWYN

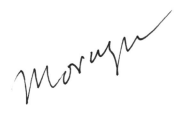

77 Lower Valley Road
West Chester, Pennsylvania 19310 USA

To Allen and Mike and the folks at the Trident Bookstore and Cafe, who kept me supplied with mochas and lattés and let me write this book there.

and

To Deborah, whose interest in all aspects of healing has been an inspiration to me.

International Standard Book Number: 0-924608-18-8
Libarary of Congress Catalog Card Number: 94-61101

Cover illustration by Steve Ferguson, Colorado Springs, CO

Published by Whitford Press
A division of Schiffer Publishing, Ltd.
77 Lower Valley Road
Atglen, PA 19310
Manufactured in the United States of America
This book may be purchased from the publisher.
Please include $2.95 postage.
Try your bookstore first.

We are interested in hearing from authors
with book ideas on related subjects.

Contents

Chapter 1:
Introduction

With the recent trends toward environmentalism, back-to-nature pursuits, alternative medicine, and the proliferation of literature on natural healing, the question springs to mind, "why another book on herbs?" Because from a Witch's point of view, much more needs to be said.

Plants are fundamental to the Witch's craft because medicinal and magical uses of herbs comprise an essential part of the philosophical construct on which the Craft is founded. Herbal medicine, also known as wortcunning, is an old and longstanding practice, and represents one of the chief points of communality among Witches of different traditions. Herbalism unites traditions as diverse as the Celtic, Egyptian, Norse, American Indian, and Qabalist.

Back in the mists of pre-recorded time, human beings struggling to survive in a hostile environment noticed that many plants in one way or another, increased human vitality. Certain ones helped stave off hunger; others provided shelter and clothing; still others healed wounds and disease. Soon it was discovered that some botanicals worked on the human organism to produce pleasure or pain, and in extreme cases, death. To primitive people, this seemed terrifying stuff.

By observing the tremendous regenerative abilities of plants in tropical climates and their remarkable cyclical habits of growth, flowering, maturation, apparent death, and resurrection in northern climes, our ancestors grew to respect and even revere the seemingly magical powers of plants.

Ancient people became nature worshippers, in part, as a response to these observations. They created the mandala of nature, or wheel of life, to explain the mysteries of life and death of which the life cycle of plants became an important symbol. Those wise women and men who understood the secrets of botanicals became the exalted spiritual leaders of ancient tribes.

Their mastery over flowers, herbs, roots, stems, leaves and buds, which they transformed into teas, oils, medicine, salves, incenses, and sachets was invaluable to the survival of the human tribe and to the improved quality of life among emerging civilizations. Plants were held in such high regard that Alchemists attempted to discover deep within their essences the key to the elixir of life; that is, the secrets of life and immortality.

As societies evolved and the medical community grew in prominence, the Shamans' bases of power gradually eroded. Soon they were debased as necromancers, sorcerers, and Witches. Their ancient wisdom was denigrated as useless superstition. And so, the search for the ineffable "elixir of life" was consigned to the trash heap as one more baseless myth of a lesser evolved people. Unfortunately, this is the state in which the magical arts remained until the twentieth century.

Many people do not understand the link between Witchcraft and herbalism. One of my friends skeptical of the Craft recently challenged me about my beliefs. He could not see why I wanted to dust off all these musty, seemingly illogical traditions that did not appear to have any significance for contemporary life. I realized that his well-meaning criticism was based on naive ideas which he had picked up from the sensationalist press, Hollywood, and irresponsible religious zealots. Such critics claim that Witchcraft is a conglomeration of folk superstitions which are out-of-date in our scientific age.

This shallow approach has no relevance to contemporary Witchcraft. The principles affirmed by modern day Witches are a far cry from antiquated superstitions. One of the distinct features of Wicca is the flexibility of its precepts, which are adaptable to the demands of different situations over time.

In the 1960's, a back-to-nature, environmentally conscious movement emerged. The adherents of this movement advocated a return to a way of life more in keeping with the natural rhythms of the earth and cosmos. Such a lifestyle enables a person to search for life's meaning in terms that supercede mere material aims. Long ago, Witches incorporated harmony with nature and personal equilibrium into their belief system. Knowledge of herbs and other plants as natural healing agents is just one manifestation of these tenets.

An allied trend particularly visible in the U.S., is a renewed interest in the subcultures of ethnic groups. As people search for an identity in their ethnic roots, they uncover valuable folk wisdom from cultures that enjoy a close relationship with nature. Native American Indian, Neo-African, and Oriental cultures are prime examples of such ethnic sub-cultures. Many of these traditions, particularly those dealing with herbal medicine and lore, have been incorporated into Wicca doctrine because the values coincide with, and deepen Witches' understanding of their own beliefs.

"Still," my friend counters, "aren't these folk healing techniques a bit artless and archaic?" Not really. The Witch's commitment to healing by using knowledge and techniques accumulated over time never goes out of style. To labor for the physical, mental, and spiritual well-being of everything on earth should be one of everybody's main goals.

As for the suggestion that herbal healing techniques are old-fashioned, I wonder why scientists are scurrying to comb the Amazon forest, which they call a "tropical pharmacy,"[1] before it disappears, in search of botanicals to cure AIDS and other diseases. Why are the British studying the common licorice plant as an aid to human fertility? Similarly, it would be difficult to explain away as mere superstition the phenomenal resurgence of interest in traditional herbal healing, Oriental herbalism, holistic medicine, chromotherapy, aura-reading, and other naturopathic techniques. Somebody out there must think that plants have not lost all significance.

Admittedly, Witches employ some currently unacceptable methods for curing age-old physical and spiritual ills based on natural substances that act upon the whole organism. Witches draw on alternative means to standard medicine in order to help alleviate pain. However, Wicca techniques such as meditation and visualization, are something that even the medical establishment is now just beginning to accept under the "scientific" name of biofeedback.

It is also true that the success of some Wicca healing mechanisms may be traced to the patient's belief that the cure will work. Religions around the world call something very much like this "faith healing." Because what Witches do when they perform healings cannot be gauged by our current, rather coarse scientific measurements does not mean that the results are any less effective than modern medicine.

"Nevertheless," my friend argues, "some Craft attributes for herbs are downright improbable. For instance, how can putting dried wormwood in your dresser drawers drive away evil forces? And it seems ridiculous that drinking a cup of lemon balm tea can enhance your speaking abilities."

Witches conceive of plants as part of the interconnective system of the cosmos. Long ago, this theory was named the Doctrine of Signatures, which states that everything in the universe is in some way linked to something else. Plants show their associations by manifesting a recognizable form, color, scent, habitat, etc., that connect to the human body. For example, the seaweed, bladderwrack, is composed of little sacks that resemble miniature human bladders. So this plant was prescribed to cure urinary tract infections long before scientific studies corroborated its diuretic effects. Coincidence? Perhaps.

Nowadays, Witches are well aware that herbs do not necessarily cure ailments according to the Doctrine of Signatures. Generally, their prescriptions stem from empirical studies rather than from this admittedly archaic doctrine. At the same time, Witches realize that a body of lore has evolved around the magical uses of herbs, and that peoples' beliefs have created a kind of magical reality for herbs which is now valid in its own right. When a Witch makes an herbal talisman or sachet for a patient to wear, she/he attempts to reach the source of the "dis-ease" on psychic and cosmic levels as well as on the physical plane. To this end, botanicals may be included according to their associations with the Doctrine of Signatures.

The rose offers an illustration of this theory. Over the centuries, people have believed that roses represent love in its purest, most exalted form. This symbol was adopted by many religions, including Christianity, Islam, and Buddhism. The Witch can concentrate on the hidden meaning of the rose during meditation or ritual along with other appropriate images such as colors, aromas, candles, modes of dress, deity forms, etc., to enhance the idea of love, and to make it more readily accessible.

Once the Witch's mind, imagination, soul, and spirit are imbued with the power of pure love, she can manifest this thought as a real and palpable force, and manipulate it to create changes on this plane. This is a primary goal of working Magic, this, and striving for "at-one-ment" with the universe.

Finally in this introduction I wish to address an issue that often arises when the uninitiated hear Witches talk about using herbs in spells, rituals, and enchantments. People are curious to know Witches' precise intentions when they work Magic.

Personally, my friends and acquaintances outside the Craft know me well enough to realize that as a Wicca priestess I do not spend my time throwing curses on people. Certainly Witches are not hell-bent on changing children into mice as a popular Hollywood movie purports. (*The Witches*, 1990, directed by Nicolas R. Roeg, starring Angelica Huston) They fully understand that such habits inflict very bad karma on the practitioner.

I am concerned by a more insidious type of misconceived criticism that goes something like this: "It appears that you are a group of women and men who gather together as a support group and perform rituals to get the things you want for each other."

To me, this rather reductionist definition of our aims sounds as if we go to some sort of occult shopping mall and fill our baskets with brightly packaged goodies labeled with names like "prosperity," "wealth," and "success." Most Witches do not regularly, if at all, practice their Craft in order to obtain material ends. To do so would dilute the magical force, and finally, render the Witch powerless.

Since most Witches believe their purpose on earth is to learn lessons about life, some of which may have been brought from other incarnations, and to work through karmic issues, they hesitate to make changes in their own, or anyone else's lives that would hinder them from tackling these challenges.

The Witch's intent when working with herbs in rituals, spells, potions, and philtres is primarily humanitarian. Craft doctrine urges Witches to help alleviate suffering. The only selfish benefit is that by helping others, Witches gain personal satisfaction.

Another goal Witches hope to achieve through their rites is to increase their knowledge of the cosmos, gain inner equilibrium and strength, and generally improve themselves physically, mentally, psychically and spiritually. The Witch's objective is to lead, in as far as she/he is able, the best of possible lives, in all senses of the word.

In this spirit, I wish to share with you the following accumulation of knowledge from my years in the Craft. I hope you find it useful.

About This Book

This book is organized into four parts which include information on herbs, teas, talismans, and precious stones.

The herbal chapter does not treat incenses, perfumes, sachets, and potpourris. This topic is so vast that it merits a separate volume, forthcoming under the title, *Witch's Brew: Secrets of Scents*. Also, it does not contain data on trees, which I addressed in *Web of Light: Rites for Witches in the New Age* (Whitford Press, 1993).

The link between herbs and teas is self-evident, as tea is considered an herb, and many herbal concoctions for health and magic are prescribed as teas.

The association between talismans, stones, and herbs is not as apparent. In the chapter on talismans, the emphasis is on preparation and consecration of herbal talismans. However, in order to understand how these talismans work, a general, introduction to familiarize the reader with properties, uses, and types of talismans is presented.

The topic of precious stones bridges the gap between herbs and talismans. Most Witches usually use precious stones as talismans, and consecrate and carry them in pouches along with other sacred objects. The bond between stones and herbs is that they both represent products of the earth, and therefore contain many similar attributes.

Finally, I advise you never to use the information from this book as a substitute for standard medical care. What is presented in these pages amounts to lore, often gathered from empirically unproven sources. In case of illness, always first see your doctor.

Chapter 2:
Philtres, Conjure Balls, and Witches' Flying Ointment

In times gone by, the dividing line between medicinal and magical uses of herbs was not as established as it is today. Any substance that could remedy physical as well as psychic ills was considered marvelous and magical. Clients visited their local Witch healers who addressed both physical and non-physical conditions such as improvement of their love life, working conditions, and legal status.

Witches became adept at fulfilling esoteric needs by prescribing potions. Two important types of potions that still are referred to in modern times, are aphrodisiacs and philtres. An aphrodisiac is a single herb or combinations of herbs, drugs, animal tissues, and powdered stones which when ingested, is reputed to enhance general physical desire and performance. Usually it is taken in a tea or added to wine in small, concentrated amounts. Aphrodisiacs are alleged to work because of their physical action on the human body.

Philtres, on the other hand, which are composed of much the same types of ingredients (plus body tissue, excretions, blood, and hair and nail clippings) are believed to succeed solely because of their magical associations, powers, and properties. Most philtres are concocted to procure the love of a specific person. However, some philtres allegedly promote courage, prosperity, and wreak vengeance.

Both types of magical potions enjoyed a popular reputation during the Middle Ages. Typical magical philtres contained herbal ingredients like melissa, coriander, marjoram, basil, vervain, myrtle, cinquefoil, violet, valerian, garlic, chick peas, pomegranates, hazelnuts, and white bryony. They also counted on poisonous plants like mandrake and black hellebore. Some ingredients of animal origin included dried and pulverized hair, feathers, plus chicken, dove, sparrow, and swallow parts, and the internal organs of the hare. Because minute, almost "homeopathic" amounts of these substances were introduced into wine and beer, the poisonous and noxious ingredients probably did little harm.

The high repute in which philtres were held remains firm today. They are still commodities much sought by Witches' clients. Many authors perpetuate these legends by making extravagant claims for their efficacy. For example, Grillot de Givry in *Witchcraft, Magic and Alchemy*, declares that philtres are "a powerful, dramatic motive force, easy to set working, and of the greatest utility in difficult situations."[2]

If you are interested in making your own philtres, I suggest you prepare a decoction from any appropriate powdered herbs listed in the herbal in chapter 7. I do not recommend the poisonous and animal components that were so fondly included in recipes of yesteryear. However, for curiosity's sake, here are some oldtime love recipes:

*Powdered periwinkle and earthworms - add to your lover's favorite meat dish. But if you don't want your lover to get ill, leave out the periwinkle, as it is poisonous!

*Powdered root of *Enula campana*, an orange, and ambergris mixed together with a piece of paper with the word "sheva" written on it.

*Powdered chicken heart and lavender (put in wine).

*Powdered heart of dove, womb of swallow, liver of sparrow, kidney of hare, and your own blood taken from your third finger - add a pinch to a glass of wine (yummy!).

Conjure Balls

Other popular herbal concoctions still in vogue today are conjure balls. Witches make conjure balls for many magical purposes including love, money, career, protection, legal aid, health, attraction, and psychic development.

Conjure balls are best fashioned over a wood fire, but you can bend the rules and use your stove if your home has no open fire. I advise against using a microwave as the wax can blow up. Soften a bit of wax in a pot over low heat. Add appropriate herbs and perfume oils distilled from herbs and flowers, your own nail clippings, blood, hair, and/or those of the person whom you wish to influence. Mix in a drop of food color (red for love, green for prosperity, yellow for intellect, purple for psychic development, orange for activity, blue for the law, spiritual development). As the wax firms up, roll it into a ball, and thread a piece of yarn or a ribbon through the top so you can wear the ball around your neck.

Recipes for Conjure Balls

All the following recipes require about 2 Tbs. of candlemaking wax, a pinch of each botanical, and 3 drops of each oil. Color with food coloring after the wax is melted and you have added the herbs. How many drops of coloring you add is up to how vivid you want to make the ball.

Love Ball

Damiana, marjoram, myrrh, nutmeg, acacia flowers, cardamom, benzoin powder. Oils: rose, benzoin, sandalwood, civet. Color: pink or red.

Prosperity Ball

Chamomile, peppermint, patchouly leaves, clover tops, cinnamon powder, marigold flowers. Oils: frankincense, clove, rose, bayberry. Color: green.

Psychic Self-Development Ball

Cinnamon powder, orris powder, mugwort, thyme, queen of the meadow. Oils: violet, rosemary, eugenol, wisteria. Color: violet.

Hex-Breaker Ball

Frankincense powder, myrrh powder, rosemary leaves, vervain, mistletoe leaves, hyssop. Oils: rose, myrrh, violet, verbena, vetivert. Color: yellow.

In my metaphysical supplies business, WildWood Studio, I regularly make conjure balls for customers. Here are the directions for use:

At dusk, go outside with your conjure ball. Facing east, raise your arms above your head and invoke the Great Guardians of the Eastern Gate of the Universe to protect you in your rite.

Turn to the south, and invoke the Guardians of the South in the same manner. Repeat the formula in the west and north. Visualize the Guardians facing you and growing taller and larger until they reach the sky.

Returning to the east, take your conjure ball in your left hand, and once again with arms raised, invoke the force of the deity appropriate to your purpose:

> Love - Aphrodite
> Prosperity - Jupiter
> Protection - Michael
> Psychic Self-Development - the Muses
> Better Health - Ra

As you invoke the deity, imagine the power flaming from the god/goddess form into your head, down your neck and shoulders, through your arms, and out your fingertips in a brilliant beam of white light. When you have visualized the power completely, move it from your right hand into the ball that is in your left hand. Intuitively you will know when the power has been transferred.

Thank the deity for lending power and influence to your rite. Take leave of the Guardians of each of the Quarters, facing the appropriate direction, beginning in the east. When you are finished, close the Circle.

Put the conjure ball into its bag. Keep it at your bedside, in your purse, briefcase, car, or hang it in a window. Make sure the window does not receive direct sunlight, or your ball may dissolve in a puddle of wax.

When the purpose of the ball has been fulfilled, melt it over a low fire, pour the wax into a hole in the ground, and cover it with earth. Perform a small private ritual of thanksgiving to the deity who helped you.

Witches' Flying Ointment

In your readings about the history of the Craft, you may have seen references to Witches' Flying Ointment. During the era of the Witch persecutions and trials, it generally was believed that Witches rubbed themselves with a magic ointment, and flew off to Sabbats on broomsticks. Much research has been performed to determine the probable ingredients of these ointments. If indeed, Witches did have recourse to these aids to catapult them onto psychic journeys, it is no wonder that they really believed they had flown and performed other marvelous feats. Most of the ingredients regularly mentioned are highly narcotic and poisonous.

Although Witches' Flying Ointment recipes vary, many included the following components: datura, water hemlock, hemlock, opium poppy, juniper, tobacco, saffron, henbane, deadly nightshade (belladonna), mandrake, poplar leaves, speedwell, yellow flag, sweet flag, parsley, parsnip, celery wild lettuce, cinquefoil, tormentil, monkshood, and darnel.

Such a combination of herbs, if it did not kill a person outright would produce dizziness, nausea, numbness, the sensation of flying, and increased powers of night vision. It is assumed that Witches applied these mixtures externally as ointments, and did not ingest the poisons. Even so, such concoctions would be extremely dangerous. Therefore, I do not recommend this recipe for internal consumption, and include it only as a matter of curiosity.

Chapter 3:

Tea

A fundamental part of herbal knowledge is the ability to prescribe beverage and medicinal teas for a variety of ailments. This is one point on which Witches and non-Witches can come together, because everybody is familiar with and enjoys tea.

Did you know that more people in the world drink tea than coffee? In fact, tea is almost as ubiquitous a beverage as water, and has been enjoyed by many cultures throughout the ages.

Tea History

Non-herbal tea, once called "the plant of heaven," probably originated in China, where legend has it that 5,000 years ago an emperor discovered its delights when some leaves fell into a pot of water he was boiling. In another story from India, Buddha, who kept dozing off during meditation, was so piqued that he cut off his eyelids and flung them to the ground. From where the eyelids fell sprang two tea bushes.

The history of the so-called "froth of liquid jade" is packed with political intrigue and romance. Tea has been involved in revolts and wars such as the American Revolution where the unpopular tax on tea led to the famous Boston Tea Party. The botanical has forced people to engage in illegal activities like smuggling, and brought about major tax reform in England.

Great fortunes, both legitimate and illegitimate, were amassed from tea during the days of the Yankee clippers. The first swift American tea clipper to arrive in England reclaimed two-thirds the cost of building the ship on one cargo load.

Tea predominates as the beverage of choice in Oriental cultures. The Japanese created the renowned tea ceremony, which is an elaborately stylized ritual that represents a model of politeness and spiritual grace and balance. In some Eastern countries, if a head of state does something contrary to the legislators' wishes, they may throw teacups at him![3]

After its introduction to England by a Portuguese queen in the seventeenth century[4] as a temperance drink, "the river of jade," as it was called, quickly became the preferred non-alcoholic liquid refreshment of all classes of society, despite its high price. The drink was so popular that moralists of the day, assuming that anything so good must be evil, raged against tea for drugging and debasing working class women. One British Prime Minister was so fond of his cuppa that at night he filled his hot water bottle with the steaming brew so it would never be far from reach.

What Is Tea?

Even though tea first was marketed in China, currently, only about 3% of the production for the international market originates in that country. Main tea producers are India (35%), Kenya (18%), and Sri Lanka (10.5%).[5]

Tea leaves grow on a kind of camellia bush considered exalted enough to merit its own genus name, *Thea sinensis*. The bush grows best at high altitudes in dry climates near the Equator. This is why India and Sri Lanka are substantial producers. However, tea is harvested in places as diverse as Japan, Mozambique, Papua/New Guinea, and Guatemala.

Teas are categorized as green, oolong, and black, which merely refers to how long the leaves are fermented before they are dried. Fermentation occurs when withered, partially dried leaves are spread on tables and covered with wet cloths. This process adds spice and aroma to the leaves.

Unfermented, heated leaves are called green teas, semi-fermented leaves make oolong teas, and fully fermented leaves create the familiar black teas we find in most restaurants.

Black teas are classified according to leaf size and appearance. Many people mistakenly think that Orange Pekoe (pronounced "peck-oh")is a type of tea. The term actually refers to a large leaf-tea that used to be scented with orange blossoms. Large-leaf tea is usually good quality, broken-leaf can vary from excellent to poor, small-leaf teas often are excellent. The very smallest leaves and broken leaves are called fannings and dust. These generally inferior quality leaves are reserved for tea bags.

Green teas are ranked according to leaf age, style, and size. The grades are called gunpowder, imperial, young hyson, and hyson.

The teas we drink often are blended or scented. In blending, India teas are selected for strength, Ceylon for flavor, and African varieties for color. China teas really only blend well with Darjeeling and Ceylon.

To create scented teas, tea growers add full flower blossoms during the drying process. After the tea passes through the final charcoal drying stage, the crisp flowers are removed, leaving a delicate aroma and flavor.

A wide variety of substances are used to scent teas including bergamot, chamomile, chrysanthemum, cinnamon, clove buds, fennel, gardenia, ginger, hibiscus, jasmine, lavender, lime, lychee, marigold, narcissus, nutmeg, orange, peach tree leaves, rose, saffron, vanilla bean, and violet.

Tea for Health?

Is tea any good for you? Will it kill you or cure your ills? Those who disapprove of the drink point to the high amounts of caffeine, which can aggravate high blood pressure and heart disease, and the tannic acid, strong enough to corrode metal.   Nonetheless, dieters love the brew because black and green teas contain no calories, but do have vitamins A, B complex, C, D, P, and a trace of manganese. Green tea even is alleged to help a person lose weight.

Some claim tea is healthful. In fact, one British brand, Typhoo, means "doctor" in Chinese. Cup per cup, the caffeine content is not as high as for a cup of coffee, due to the brewing process. It is claimed that since caffeine is a diuretic, it is capable of removing some poisons from the system. Caffeine also helps keep the mind active. Because tea also contains the mild muscle relaxants, theophylline and theobromine, it seems you can be relaxed, but alert, if you drink tea. Rather like having your cake and eating it too!

The tannins which give tea its taste are not the type used to tan leather. Tea's tannic acid helps the stomach digest fatty foods, and fights alkaloid poisons and other noxious bacteria. Tea even has been administered successfully in cases of nicotine and heroine withdrawal to ease the recovery process.

Studies show that people who regularly drink green or oolong tea rarely contract certain cancers.[6] The British take tea to ameliorate cold symptoms. And finally, the Chinese imbibe it to regularize systemic imbalances.

Drinking Tea

Always store tea, whether black or herbal, in an airtight container to preserve its freshness. If black tea goes stale, spread a thin layer on a sheet of paper for a few hours in a well-aired room.

Experts agree that the best way to enjoy a good cup of tea is to prepare an infusion. This consists of boiling one cupful of water, pouring it over one teaspoonful of leaves, and steeping the brew in a nonmetal container for five minutes. If you brew it in a pot, add an extra teaspoonful "for the pot," as the British say. Strain, and pour into a teacup. Add sugar, honey, or molasses if desired. Stir once, and drink while hot. Natural soft, filtered water makes a superior cup of tea.

Other Uses for Tea

Besides drinking tea you can do any of the following: combine it with sage as a hair rinse; add salt and lemon to tea, and bathe your feet in it to alleviate fungal infections and sores; dye lace, net curtains, and stockings with it; chew the leaves to get rid of bad breath or toothaches; use it as a mild disinfectant for wounds; lay cold, wet tea bags on your tired, puffy eyes to soothe them; wash your face in it to eliminate pimples; throw spent leaves, salt, and hot water into an accidentally burned saucepan, and leave overnight to remove the residue; use it as a furniture polish; cure food in its smoke; fertilize camellias with the leaves.   However you take your tea, you'll find it a refreshing, relaxing way to take a break from your daily activities.

Top Ten Teas

If you consider the kinds of tea that can be made from herbs, the number of possible blends is endless. To help you sift your way through the infinite variety of teas available at your grocery or health food store, here is a selected list of ten best sellers with a short description to accompany each.

Ceylon - grown in Sri Lanka, this brightly colored tea has a flowery aroma and light aftertaste.

Constant Comment - this recipe hails from the American South, where during Colonial times it was brewed with orange peel and clove.

Darjeeling - a full-bodied, amber-colored liquid with a pleasant taste grown at about 7,000 feet in the Himalayas.

Earl Grey - a secret formula given to a British Prime Minister by a Chinese mandarin in gratitude for having saved his life. It contains black China and Darjeeling teas scented with bergamot.

English Breakfast - a delightfully mellow, full-bodied blend of Indian and Ceylon teas that will start your day out right.

Formosa Oolong - an expensive blend of partially fermented China teas scented with peach blossoms.

Gunpowder - this green tea is named for the grayish-green color of the young leaves that resemble powder pellets.

Irish Breakfast - a medium-strong blend of black teas guaranteed to jolt you awake in the morning.

Keemun - formerly known as the traditional China imperial tea, it has a spicy bouquet. However, the quality can vary depending on the year's harvest.

Russian Caravan - in times gone by, this strong blend of China teas was packed into bricks for easy transport and carried over the steppes by caravans to Moscow.

Herbal Teas

"Herbal Tea brings pleasant dreams
Beauty, health and wealth, it seems"
Mitzie Stuart Keller[7]

Herbal teas have been brewed for centuries both as tasty beverages and medicinal agents. In fact, Chinese medicine is in part, based on prescribing medicinal teas. Herbal teas act more subtly and gently on the system than standard medicine, and address the whole body rather than just the symptoms of the disease. However, while the effects of many herbs are mild, others can be highly narcotic, intoxicating, and deadly. For instance, a tea concocted from a poisonous plant such as water hemlock, will kill you.

Herbal teas benefit a person by providing small amounts of essential vitamins and minerals. They also stimulate or suppress the appetite, settle the stomach, control the bowels, ease symptoms of colds and flu, cleanse and purify the system, act as a tonic, stimulate or relax the body, and alleviate a potpourri of ills from blood pressure problems to venereal diseases.

The American colonists valued the benefits of herbal teas, and used them as medicine when standard treatment was unavailable. So, when taxing of black tea ranged out of control the people naturally turned to these teas to help them foil the British. They substituted herbs like four-leaved loosestrife, chicory, sage, melissa, currant and raspberry leaves, and Labrador tea. The resourceful colonists even brewed a kind of tea from oven-browned field corn!

Tasty Herbal Teas

To prepare your own beverage blends, choose two or three plants from the following list (or from herbs recommended in Chapter 7). Use the leaves and flowers only. Also go to the grocery or health food store and study the ingredients' labels of your favorite herbal teas. This will give you a sense of compatible flavors. Don't forget that you also can flavor black teas with herbs and flowers.

Popular Herbal Tea Ingredients

Agrimony, alfalfa, aniseed, basil, bee balm, betony, borage, celery seed, chamomile flowers, chicory, red clover blossom, coltsfoot, dandelion leaves and root, elder flowers, eyebright, fennel, feverfew, golden rod, golden seal, horehound, hyssop, lavender flowers, marjoram, meadowsweet, nettle, peppermint, persimmon leaves, plantain, rose petals, rosemary, rue (use only a pinch—it's bitter), sage, sarsparilla, sassafrass root, spearmint, strawberry leaves, tansy, thyme, violet, yarrow flowers.

Preparing Medicinal Teas

Prepare herbal medicinal tea somewhat differently from herbal beverage or black teas. Add two to three fresh sprigs or two dried teaspoonfuls of herbs to 1-1/2 cups cold water (or white wine). Boil for ten minutes, and simmer for five more minutes until the liquid is reduced by one-third. This makes an infusion (see Appendix I.) Use only flowers and leaves for infusions.

Boil and simmer for twice the time, and you get a decoction (see Appendix I.) Use stems and roots for decoctions.

Brew beverage teas as you would black teas. Use half the amount of herbs you would for an infusion, and twice as many fresh herbs as dried.

A great way to have fresh, healthy, tasty teas is to pick your own botanicals. If you do not own an herb garden, and are gathering in the wild, make sure you do not harvest herbs that have been doused with pesticides. And never pick more than one-third of the available herbs to give them a chance to regenerate. Take along a plant identification book with pictures to avoid poisonous plants.

Medicinal Tea Herbs

The following list shows typical medicinal herbs that make good infusions and decoctions, and their action on the body. Other herbs used for tea can be found in the Witch's Herbal in chapter 7.

agrimony - for chills, fever.
alfalfa - for weight loss (combine with fennel and guaraná).
angelica - aromatic stimulant; suppresses flatulence; a tonic against nausea.
aniseed - for colds.
basil - settles the stomach.
bayberry - use a decoction for severe menstrual bleeding.
betony - a nervine, parasiticide, and alterative; substitute for black tea.
bistort - for diarrhea.
borage - mix with lemon, sugar, and wine to cure sore throats and restore strength after an illness.
cascara sagrada - a laxative.
catnip - a relaxant; for nervous headaches and children's diarrhea; combine with melissa and marshmallow root to help cure childrens' colic and colds.
chamomile - a sopophoric; stimulates the digestion; the German variety helps suppress the appetite.
chicory - a liver tonic and diuretic.
cinquefoil - for diarrhea.
coltsfoot - an expectorant.
damiana - an alleged aphrodisiac.
dandelion - a diuretic and blood tonic; settles the stomach; increases mother's milk.
dill - settles the stomach.
echinancea- a lymphatic cleanser.
fennel - an appetite suppressant.
feverfew- promotes menstruation; good for colds, diarrhea.
gentian - a stimulant, digestive, and tonic.

ginger - quells stomach trouble and motion sickness; a cold soother.
ginseng - a glandular balancer and energizer.
golden seal - for infections.
hibiscus - soothes the digestive tract.
hops - a nervine, sedative, anondyne, and tonic.
horehound - for colds and sore throat.
hyssop - antiasthmatic; an infusion loosens phlegm.
kava-kava root - a diuretic, tonic, nervine, analgesic, and sedative,
        (don't overdo, as it's narcotic!).
lemon balm - an antispasmodic, sedative, and tonic; regulates and
        brings on menses; quells stomach cramps, poor digestion,
        colic, nausea, sore throat; brings down fevers; increases urine.
licorice - a demulcent, blood purifier, expectorant, laxative, and
        alterative; soothes coughs, colds, intestinal troubles, ulcers,
        stress disorders; a female hormone balancer; promotes fertil-
        ity.
marjoram - settles the stomach.
marshmallow root - a demulcent; good for internal inflammations.
meadowsweet - a diuretic and tonic; a diet tea; suppresses diarrhea;
        an ingredient in some aspirin.
motherwort - a sedative; brings on menses; calms heart palpita-
        tions.
mullein - for coughs and swollen glands.
nettles - an alterative and tonic; drink it to lose weight; a blood
        coagulant; helps the body assimilate minerals, so it treats
        anemia.
peppermint - an antispasmodic, disinfectant, and nervine; excellent
        for colds, flu, insomnia, toothache, rheumatism sore throat,
        headache and stomachache.
raspberry leaves - an antispasmodic and stimulant; for female disor-
        ders.
rose hips - an emmenagogue, stomachic, and laxative; increases
        semen, quells vomiting, high in vitamin C.
saffron - a diaphoretic, emmenagogue, and hemostatic that stops
        uterine hemorrhages.
sage - an antispasmodic, antipyretic, carminative, and stimulant;
        slows night sweats and post nasal drip; drink for headaches,
        tonsillitis, and kidney troubles; it makes a fine sore throat
        gargle.

savory - settles the stomach.

skullcap - an antipyretic, antispasmodic, nervine, and tonic; it helps
in cases of convulsions, neuralgia, coughs, headaches, alcohol
withdrawal symptoms, and sterility; a nerve tonic and
calmative.

senna - a laxative.

solomon's seal - alleviates dysentery; a restorative tonic for stomach
and bowels.

strawberry leaves - an anti-abortive, diuretic, laxative, and female
tonic.

yarrow - an anti-inflammatory, diaphoretic, antibacterial, antipyretic,
carminative, hemostatic, mild stimulant, and vulnerary.

yerba santa - an astringent, expectorant, stomachic, and bitter tonic;
good for head colds.

yellow dock - an alterative, mild tonic, nutritive, cholagogue, and
laxative; acts against jaundice, rheumatism, and skin diseases.

Occult Uses of Herbal Teas

Naturally, since herbs constitute an important part of folk medicine, many alleged occult uses for herbs have evolved. The next list
details the supposed effects of some of the herbs most widely used
for Magic, and also are commonly found in health food stores or the
grocery. Other uses are detailed in chapter 7. Often the tea is not
meant to be drunk, but is applied as a floorwash, bath, or to sprinkle
around a room to purify it. Unless otherwise directed, use one teaspoonful of the dried herb to one cup of water.

alfalfa - grants a youthful appearance; insures against poverty.

anise - psychic development; enlivens the passions.

basil - an aphrodisiac; brings success to a business and keeps evil
away from home (floorwash).

bistort - wards off poltergeists (floorwash).

black cohosh - sprinkle around the ritual area for protection, or
around the bed at night so quarrelling couples will reconcile.

blessed thistle - brings blessings on all planes.

burdock - cleanses and purifies the ritual area.

catnip - drives away nightmares.

chamomile - rinse your hands in the tea before beginning the business day to attract customers; also rinse your hands in the tea to which you have added 9 drops of gamblers' perfume oil to win at games of chance.

cinnamon - attracts love.

clove -attracts love.

clover - brings prosperity.

coriander -attracts love and keeps your mate from wandering.

damiana - an aphrodisiac; steep in boiling water, and put some in your lover's food so she/he will always be yours.

dandelion - to summon spirits, drink a cup before retiring, and leave a steaming bowl of the brew by your bedside; add it to coffee to protect yourself from disease; drink it to overcome despondency.

dill - an aphrodisiac.

dulse - promotes friendship and happiness.

elecampane - an aphrodisiac; use in beauty spells.

eyebright - promotes prophetic dreams; aids concentration in rituals.

fennel - confers strength; invokes Diana.

fenugreek - combine this tea and lemon verbena oil in a floor wash to draw cash.

feverfew - drink it to stay healthy and avoid stress.

five fingers grass - removes curses and hexes (bath).

hops - for astral travel and protection.

hyssop - for meditation and ritual (bath).

kelp - wash church floors with the tea to attract parishioners.

lady's mantle - for female fertility.

lemon balm - drink before speaking in public, as it is said to rejuvenate the mind and body; relieves melancholy.

life everlasting - drink daily for a long, happy life.

lovage - calms your nerves and those of all with whom you come in contact (bath).

marshmallow - 1 ounce to 1 gallon of water steeped for nine days and added to child's bath will protect her/him.

meadowsweet - 1 teaspoon to 1 pint of water added to bath will help you obtain employment and improve your clairvoyance; if you drink this tea, good fortune will smile on all your endeavors.

motherwort - in Japan, drinking this tea is said to increase the lifespan.

mugwort - for divination; it is poisonous if ingested in large amounts.

peppermint - for prophetic dreams, drink at bedtime; a purification water for rituals.

queen root - to get pregnant.

rose - sprinkle the tea on your bed to revitalize love; an old Burmese custom is to brew a tea with sandalwood and rosewater and bathe in it at the New Year to wash away the sins of the old year — only don't drink it, as sandalwood is poisonous.

rue - for clairvoyance.

saffron - a sexual stimulant.

Saint Johnswort - 1 ounce herb to 1 quart water in a decoction and used as a floorwash will drive out evil; as you wash the floor, say, "St. John, into Thy hands, I place my welfare."

senna - steep for seven days 1 tablespoon in 1 quart of water, and anoint your lover's thighs with it so she/he will never be able to offer favors to another.

slippery elm - sprinkle around the house as a peace water.

solomon's seal - use in exorcisms.

snake root - a decoction in a bottle steeped for seven days and spread on the soles of your shoes will lead you to money.

spikenard - anoint the picture of a loved one with a decoction of this root to encourage lifelong fidelity.

lemon verbena - drink or use in the bath to be successful in the arts; an ingredient of holy water.

vervain - wash your hands and the people you touch will be attracted to you; vervain washwater protects the house and brings wishes home to roost.

yarrow - dispels melancholy.

yellow dock - wash the doorknobs of your business or house with the tea to bring good fortune.

Zodiac Tea Recipes

The following zodiac tea recipes include edible botanicals from each sun sign chosen to strengthen the characteristics of the sign. As I also do with zodiac oils, I include something from the opposite sign to help balance the personality. For example, Leo tea will include one Aquarius botanical. Mix together equal parts of each botanical unless otherwise indicated. Make an infusion by steeping a teaspoon of the mixture in one cup of steaming water for five minutes. Filter and drink once a day to fortify yourself.

Aries: 1/4 nettle, 1 peppermint, 1/2 watercress, 1/2 hops, golden seal (pinch).
Taurus: 1/2 dandelion leaves, 1/4 dandelion root, 1/4 lovage, 1/8 horehound, 1/8 fennel seed.
Gemini: 1/2 meadowsweet, 1/4 parsley, 1/4 caraway seed, vervain (pinch).
Cancer: 1/4 honeysuckle flowers, 1 lemon balm, 1/4 violet leaves, 1/2 comfrey, hyssop (pinch).
Leo: 1 peppermint, 1/2 chamomile, 1/4 angelica root, 1/4 fennel, 1/4 anise.
Virgo: 1/2 fennel seed, 1/4 rosemary, 1 peppermint, 1/4 whole cloves, ground cloves (pinch), 1/4 marjoram, 1/4 skullcap.
Libra: 1/2 strawberry leaves, 1/4 catnip, 1/4 violet leaves, 1/2 watercress, marjoram (pinch).
Scorpio: 1/4 horehound, 1/4 basil, 1 lovage, 1/2 sarsparilla, 1 raspberry leaves, 1/4 parsley.
Sagittarius: 1/2 chicory (roasted root), 1/2 wood betony, 1/4 vervain, golden seal (pinch).
Capricorn: 1/2 linden, 1 lemon balm, 1/2 peppermint, 1/4 comfrey, hyssop (pinch).
Aquarius: 1/4 spikenard, 1/2 strawberry leaves, 1/4 fennel, 1/2 eyebright, 1/2 peppermint.
Pisces: 1/4 peppermint, 1/2 chamomile flowers, 1/4 wood betony, 1/4 Irish moss, 1/2 elder flowers, agrimony (pinch).

Tea Leaf Reading

Start reading someone's tea leaves, and I guarantee you'll soon draw a crowd. Everybody wants to know what the future will bring, and tea leaf reading is an easily accessible, relatively uncomplicated, light-hearted way to practice divination. In a word, tea leaves are user-friendly.

Every object we touch faintly records the energy emitted by our auras, and tea leaves seem particularly impressionable. William Hewitt in *Tea Leaf Reading* claims that since every cell in our bodies contains all the past, present and future information about us, the

pattern left by tea leaves will express some of this personal information.[8]

The way tea leaves show this information is by clinging together
to form easily decipherable images that are left on the sides and
bottom of the cup after the tea is drunk. These pictures can be interpreted either literally or symbolically as snapshots of the future of the
person who has consumed the tea.

The influenceablilty of tea leaves is only strong enough to pick up
data from the past, present, or near future. Yet within this range, the
information they reveal is extremely accurate.

Another joy of tea leaf reading is that unlike other forms of
divination like the tarot and crystal gazing, years of meditation are
not required to perfect your technique. All you need is a dollop of
imagination, a pinch of intuition, the ability to memorize meanings of
symbols, and a storyteller's gift, and you're in business.

The Teacup

All right, you want to be a tea leaf reader for fun, profit, or in a
sincere desire to help people achieve their highest potential. How do
you go about it? First, choose a cup.   It must be a real teacup, not a
mug. White porcelain is best because it clearly shows leaf patterns.
Transparent cups, or cups with designs on the inside are not practical
because they distract the reader and distort impressions. Cups with
high vertical sides or small openings at the top will cause the leaves
to bunch up, which makes them difficult to read.

A perfect cup is one that slopes outward from the base. Some
readers prefer square cups because they find it easy to pinpoint
events using the corners as a frame of reference.

Preparing for a Reading

Next comes the easy part: find someone who'll let you read his or
her leaves, whom we will call the "inquirer." The inquirer should
prepare her/his own cup of tea whenever possible to instill the tea
with personal vibrations. If this is inconvenient, instruct the inquirer
to hold cupped palms over the prepared cup for a few minutes,
concentrating all the while on her/his personal hopes, dreams and
challenges.

Use loose leaves, either black, green, or herbal. The fannings and dust that make up tea bags may not produce clear images.

If you are reading for a specific question, choose a theme tea, like peppermint for money, rosehips for love, chamomile for health and success. If you select Constant Comment or a scented tea like jasmine, the flowers and peels will incorporate into the reading, and create interesting images.

Coarse teas tend produce a few bold images that are ideal for short readings. Finer teas render more numerous, complex designs, often showing one large figure and several smaller groupings. These images are good for an inquirer who has many questions or a busy life. Interestingly, the same tea will produce diverse picture styles for different people.

Place one-half teaspoonful of dried, black leaves, or one teaspoonful of fresh herbs in a cup, and pour boiling water over the leaves. Stir once to distribute the leaves evenly, and steep for five minutes before drinking. Do not add sweetener or milk because they make sticky leaves that do not lie naturally on the sides of the cup.

Place the cup on a saucer with a napkin between them, and have a spoon ready so you can point to the formations you see. This is interesting to the inquirer, and helps lend credence to your reading.

Do a preliminary scan by examining the surface of the water. Bubbles mean a monetary windfall. Sticks floating on top of the water presage visitations. A long, thin stick stands for a woman; a short, fat stick for a man.

Tell the inquirer to place hands over the cup, make a wish, and leisurely drink all but about one teaspoonful of the liquid. Now, the inquirer gently rotates the cup, swirling the liquid around, and tips it more and more until it trickles out evenly, and the cup is inverted over the napkin on the saucer. The napkin minimizes messes by absorbing the liquid.

This slow inversion method is a bit tricky, and some people may not feel up to it. If your inquirer balks, have her/him invert the cup over the napkin all at once, and turn the cup clockwise three times before setting it on the saucer. Some leaves inevitably are lost with either method. Once, when I was giving a tea leaf reading class, a student asked me, "What if all the leaves fall out?" I replied quickly, "That never happens." She inverted her cup, and naturally, all the leaves came dribbling out. So we read the saucer!

After five minutes, you, the reader, pick up the cup, and daub up any excess water without dislocating the leaves. No water residue should remain in the cup, but if there is, by tradition, each drop represents a tear the inquirer will shed.

Reading the Leaves

Now it is your turn to examine the leaves. Relax; take your time. Pretend you are lying on your back reading cloud formations. Never force an image. Just let them flow into your consciousness.

Look for concrete, realistic shapes like faces, people, animals, trees, and flowers, and familiar objects like cars, houses, furniture, etc. Check out the cup for geometrical forms like triangles, circles, squares, dots, and straight lines.

Go on to numbers, letters, and spelled-out words. Note standard symbols like crosses, stars, and signs of the zodiac. Look for single images and groups of images.

Make a general assessment of the pictures you find. How many are positive? how many negative? Bigger figures may carry more weight than smaller ones. Although the pictures are usually symbolic, sometimes they may refer to exactly what they depict. For instance, a dog may indicate the inquirer's dog.

Examine the cup from all angles, even upside down. Sometimes you'll find two figures in the same grouping by viewing it from different angles. Both signs are valid, and they are linked. If symbols fall within a quarter inch of each other, interpret them as mutually influential. Trust your first impressions, and use common sense.

Throughout the reading, stress the positive. If you say, "Gosh, I see you falling down a staircase next month and injuring yourself badly," your inquirer surely will be talked into doing just that. Perhaps it is better to suggest, "In about a month you might take care around staircases to avoid possibly slipping. If you are mindful, you will be fine." After all, the inquirer is coming to you to find out what may happen, not what necessarily will happen. Everyone has the free will to change the probable course of events laid out by the reader. This is why people have readings in the first place.

There are three ways to ascertain when events will take place. In one method, signs near the rim show occurrences that will take place sooner than those near the bottom. Events at the bottom happen after three or four months.

By another method, symbols that face the handle mean approaching events, while those facing away indicate departing influences.

In the third way, the handle represents present time, and leaves grouped around it show what will occur within the next few days, or alternatively, the inquirer's personality traits that will affect the events of the timespan.

Moving clockwise around the cup, one quarter of the way is one month, one-half is two months, three-quarters, three months, and back to the right side of the handle shows four months. Events close to the rim will happen at the beginning of a month, those in the middle, toward the middle of a month, and those toward the bottom, but not directly on the bottom, will transpire at the end of a given month.

In this system, images at the bottom of the cup are valid throughout the entire four-month span. However, in my experience, I have come to believe that what remains at the bottom of the cup may not necessarily represent actual occurrences, but emotional, physical, and spiritual effects of events on the inquirer.

Some symbols contain more than one meaning. A fence may refer to property or constriction of one's freedom. A cat can be taken to mean a jealous person or development of psychic potential. A figure of a woman may stand for an acquaintance, happiness, or the zodiac sign, Virgo. Some readers recommend never to interpret a sign literally.

Others prefer to call a breadbox a breadbox only if it is linked with a number or letter. I think how you explain a sign depends very much on the other images in the cup and your own gut feeling.

Look for nearby figures to help you understand a symbol. A star by itself may mean success or inspiration. Coupled with a dancer, for example, it may signify accomplishment in the arts. Linked to a book, the inquirer may soon study astrogeophysics or a related field.

The phase where you contemplate the cup should only last for about five minutes, or your inquirer may grow impatient or anxious. With practice, you soon will be able to elicit the significant symbols from the cup quickly.

Keep a list of your personal interpretations of symbols. You may not always agree with standard definitions. For example, a frog is supposed to signify a drastic change or move, probably because frogs take sudden leaps. However, for me, the frog is a symbol of both physical and mental creativity and fertility. A list of some common symbols and their interpretations is in Appendix II. Other symbols and their significance for tea leaf reading are detailed elsewhere in this book. Constantly strive to broaden your scope by leafing through symbol dictionaries. *A Dictionary of Symbols* by J.E. Cirlot is one that I have found helpful.

You are ready to weave your story. Tea leaf reading should be fun for both the inquirer and you. So tell an engaging story based on the evidence. Building a strong narrative from the signs lends coherence and continuity to your reading. Interpreting symbols without a structure can leave the inquirer with a fuzzy impression. Place together coupled events, pay attention to the timeframe references, and the effects on the inquirer shown at the bottom of the cup.

You also can give a past life reading, or a reading to answer a specific question. In these cases, time referencing does not apply. Someone might like a past life reading to find out what prior events have influenced current conditions.

While the tea leaves can consider specific questions, they are not as adept at yes/no questions as other modes of divination like the pendulum. If an inquirer has a specific question, ask him, when placing his hands over the cup, to concentrate on the question from all possible angles. This will give a truer reading.   Tea leaf reading is an entertaining and enriching experience for both the inquirer and the reader. So, I raise my cup of Earl Grey to you in a toast, and wish you good luck!

Chapter 4:

Precious Stones:
An Occult Lapidary

Perhaps because human beings are largely composed of minerals, or because stones represent our origin and home on Mother Earth, or maybe it is on account of their aesthetic qualities. For whatever reason, the beauty of stones is often compared to that of flowers, but the seduction of flowers seems ephemeral when compared to the elegance of stones. In human terms, while flowers are compared to the emotions, stones are likened to the gifts of the spirit.

Attraction to the sparkling, variegated beauty of precious stones is a fascination common to all cultures throughout history. Ancient people interpreted the association of the spirituality of stones literally, and believed in spirits who made their homes in every rock and who represented some aspect of the divinity. The Chinese and Japanese, who sought in the great age and stark beauty of rocks a symbol of spiritual insight, and wisdom, placed unusual rocks in their gardens to aid their meditations. Similarly, Witches employ stones as points of energy concentration for focusing and directing the will.

Objections to Stone Magic

People who are not involved with Magic can raise some strong, often perfectly justifiable objections to Witches' and Magicians' use of stones. They point to the mass of misinformation currently being disseminated by some adherents of the New Age gem fad. For example, many enthusiasts assert that quartz and other minerals emit energy which cannot be physically measured. They often describe this energy as a "vibration," or "light."

Such statements are untrue, assert detractors, because all stones are physically stable and chemically inert with the exception of radioactive minerals. They cannot conduct an electric current. The only feat some minerals can perform is to develop a static charge when acted upon by an outside energy force. Remove the outside power source, and the mineral once again becomes inert. This phenomenon is known as piezoelectricity.

Gemologists and geologists also deprecate the wild, unfounded claims made by amateurs uneducated in the basic physical principles of stones that the figmental vibratory powers of stones can cure a collection of maladies from AIDS to zits.

I agree with the detractors as to gem healers' radical ideas about the abilities of most stones to physically cure disease. Unfortunately, such wishful thinking can cause real physical harm if a patient relies exclusively on gem therapy. Also I believe that the all too prevalent, lazy approach to the study of rocks results in naive, misguided notions handed down as gospel to the even less knowledgeable.

How Witches Use Stones in Magic

However, not all of us who work with stones are ignorant, and many healers who use them in Magic can achieve admirable results.

Stones are beneficial in meditation. The myriad of lovely colors and shapes imply endless themes for meditation, not least of which is the link between stones and the environment, and the need to preserve the earth. Other subjects often are suggested by the magical symbolism of the colors, which represent ideas about love, money, career, emotion, etc.

Such concepts can be introduced into rituals, where Witches charge an appropriate stone with a psychic force to bring about changes in consciousness. The changes with which the Witch instills the rock, are immeasurable by physical means that science has perfected up to now, and may not even be of the physical plane—impossible to prove, except by the results that are obtained. In short, the psychological effects of stones can be as effective as any other talisman, and therefore, should be studied with respect.

The topaz is an example of a healing gemstone. This stone is related to leadership and wisdom, so a Witch would use it in a ritual to attract these forces. Topaz is perceived to embody the essence of these qualities because over time, people have believed that it does. Unconsciously a powerful thought form has been created in association with this stone that envelops this energy.

According to Witches and other Occultists, a thought form exists by virtue of the creative power of the collective mind.

The stone itself has no power, but its presence at a ritual represents the link by which the Witch can merge her/his will with the thought-form, and direct it for a specific purpose. In simple terms, thoughts become reality because the Witch wills them to be so.

A third way in which Witches practice Stone Magic is to look into the past and divine the future. Witches believe that everything absorbs impressions of other objects and forces that exist in the environment. Stones and tea leaves seem to retain more than their fair share of influences. This does not mean that objects physically absorb and retain images like we do in our brains because we have nerves and synapses. Frankly, I cannot speculate on how this happens; I have no scientific explanation. I only can say that all objects, including stones, seem to retain these pictures, and that a sensitive person, known as a psychometrist, can hold these items and receive visual, auditory, and emotional thoughts about them, including age, origin, and surrounding events.

I have witnessed psychometrists work with police departments, and relay accurate information about which they could have no prior knowledge. Their findings often have led to the capture and conviction of criminals, finding missing persons, and solving crimes. Some psychometrists specialize in psychically unlocking information from stones that somehow "witnessed" ancient cultures and ways of life.

Other Occultists use stones, particularly quartz and precious gems, to predict the future. The stone becomes a tool for concentration in much the same way as for meditation (for a complete description of divination by crystals, see *Secrets of a Witch's Coven*).

Choosing and Charging Stones

When you select a stone for a particular magical purpose, use your intuition to pick the one that feels best to you. No stone is pure in its characteristics. Two tourmalines, for example, will vary in the amounts of other minerals they contain. Sometimes the color, feel, or shape of a gem may be more important than its composition, because the sensory impact of one will reach your subconscious mind more readily than another.

As with all magical tools, store your stones in a dark and private place, like a closet, chest, or drawer, and wrap them in dark-colored silk or cotton. If you leave them for the whole world to observe, handle, and influence, they will quickly lose their personal significance, and consequently, their magical efficacy.

Exorcise extraneous psychic influences, and personalize your stone by purifying and consecrating it to your will. First clean and polish it. Then open a Circle, and pass the stone through the symbols of the four elements: incense (for air - use Purification, Temple Rite, or Consecration incense), candle flame for fire, consecrated water, and salt for earth. The talismanic ritual in Chapter 6 shows one way to consecrate a stone.

Appendix III summarizes the composition of many common stones. You may wish to select stones according to color rather than composition, especially if you use the Doctrine of Signatures.

The following lapidary details many common stones used in Magic, and names their rulers. This is important if you are performing a planetary rite. Planetary rites are probably the most commonly attempted rituals in Magic. Both magical and curative uses of stones are described. I cannot recommend the use of gems in physical healing, but include these references as a matter of curiosity. Also you can use this information as a focus for psychic healing.

Stone Colors

According to the Doctrine of Signatures, stones, like botanicals are linked to the human body. Their virtues are believed to manifest mainly through color. I offer the old meanings of stones in healing because of the psychological value placed on them, which in turn, can be used in Magic.

RED

Red stones are believed to affect general health, the heart, blood circulation, and sex. Red promotes activity, and allegedly increases energy, heals wounds, stops bleeding, diminishes fevers and cramps, and draws poisons to surface of skin.
Stones: ruby, jasper, carnelian, bloodstone, almandine, spinel ruby, rhondonite, garnet, agate, magnetite.

PINK

A lighter variation of red, pink arouses innocent love and the sense of joy remembered from childhood. Gem healers believe that the color works on the thymus gland and encourages creative thinking.
Stones: rose quartz, coral.

ORANGE

Orange stones are said to stimulate the alimentary tract, spleen, and pancreas. They supposedly dissolve gall and kidney stones, enhance self-image, and nullify the effects of long-term illnesses. Perhaps gem healers believe these stones work on the digestive system because it is proven that orange-colored food best stimulates the appetite.[9]
Stones: orange jacinth, orange carnelian, fire opal, heliodor, topaz.

GOLD

Because of its association with the sun, gold is alleged to strengthen the heart, act as an antispasmodic, and restore self- confidence.
Stones: cat's eye, tiger's eye, gold topaz, chrysoberyl, pyrite, sunstone.

YELLOW

A color linked to the intellect, beginnings, and the direction east, yellow stones are thought to influence the brain, nerves, intelligence, speaking abilities, and communication. According to gem healers, these stones also attract hydrogen, that somehow combats indigestion and fortifies tissues, and influences the liver, solar plexus, skin, and nerves. Yellow gems are said to help cure diabetes, leprosy, and fatigue. Used in meditation, they help the dreamer achieve goals.
Stones: citrine, topaz, yellow diamond, yellow sapphire, yellow carnelian.

GREEN

The psychological effects of the color green help increase a person's sense of balance, self-control, maturity, judgment, and esthetics. Clear, green stones, when contemplated during meditation, act to refine one's inner vision. Olive, khaki, pine, yellow, and pea-green shades cultivate cheerfulness, practicality, economy, and a sense of sociability and hospitality.

Gem healers attest that green stones attract helium, and employ them in cases of ailments concerning the heart, kidneys, eyes, cerebellum, female organs, and stomach. They are believed to rid the patient of influenza, neuralgia, migraine, cancer, venereal disease, and high blood pressure.
Stones: nephrite, emerald, olivine, chrysolite, peridot, aventurine, serpentine, jade, alexandrite.

BLUE

True blue has been demonstrated to calm the mind, induce sleep, lower blood pressure and vitality, and facilitate abstinence, sobriety, and good hygiene.

Gem healers believe that these stones attract oxygen to the body and consequently, help form red blood cells. They consider these stones antiseptic and disinfectant, and use them as a cure for abscesses, ulcers, fever, dysentery, cholera, stings, hemorrhages, menstrual pain, nervous headaches, insomnia, heart palpitations, and sore throat.

Stones: blue sapphire, lapis, sodalite, azurite, galenite, moonstone, labradonite, blue calcite.

Peacock blue can irritate sensitive people and induce recalcitrant and hyper-critical behavior. However, it is a stimulating color for an unconventional and individualistic thinker.

Stones: turquoise, malachite, amazonite, aquamarine.

Indigo intensifies clairvoyance, clairaudience, and psychometric abilities, and mitigates pain, and the effects of mental illness, fits, delirium tremens, hypochondria, hallucinations, and hysteria.

Stones: spinel ruby, pyrope, lapis lazuli.

BROWN

Brown stabilizes, revives, and consoles. It is a good stone for those who are impressionable, imaginative, or reckless, because it helps balance the desires.

Stones: topaz, agate, sardonyx, carnelian.

WHITE

A combination of all colors, gem healers allege that white stones increase lactation, and strengthen and cleanse the etheric body.

Stones: white chalcedony, white serpentine, white agate, opal.

BLACK

The absence of color is known as black, and is conducive to abstract thought, self-control, and steadiness. Black stones help a person increase inner strength in the face of reversals.
Stones: jet, obsidian, onyx.

An Occult Lapidary

AGATE
Rulers: Gemini, Virgo, Cancer.

Agate is an opaque silicon dioxide quartz or chalcedony that forms concentric layers. It displays a diversity of colors and patterns. A common pattern is called moss agate, or mocha stone which is made when bubbles or other materials enter the stone in its formative stages. The stone is named for the Achates river where it was first found in abundance.

According to myth, agate sharpens the wits and sight, and enhances one's inherent gracefulness. It is an alleged antidote to poison, especially snakebite. In former times, foodtasters drank from goblets made from agate, jacinth, malachite, or topaz.

The ancients wore agate to help them polish their conversational skills, fortify them against temptation, increase their receptivity, vitality, and courage, and drive away storms.

Orpheus took agate with him to Hades to placate the gods. The stone is said to help the wearer discover treasures and gain inheritance.

Black agate keeps enemies away, makes athletes victorious in competition, and brings luck to gamblers. The red variety defends the wearer from lightning, and brings peace and protection. The blue-laced type is said to be the most compatible with "little-girl" energy. Brown agate confers wealth and a long, happy life, while the green-colored stone supposedly cures eye afflictions and enhances female fertility. The botswana patterned agate brings good news and small pleasures.

ALEXANDRITE

Ruler: Gemini.

This stone was named for Alexander II of Russia, because it was discovered on his birthday. It is a green chrysoberyl containing chromium, but no silica. Alexandrite appears red or reddish-purple in candlelight.

It is used by gem healers and Magicians like all green stones, and is said to be particularly effective in consolidating personal power by strengthening the aura.

AMBER

Rulers: Sun, Leo.

Amber is not an actual stone, but a petrified resin of extinct conifer trees. However, it is mounted like a gem in jewelry. Both clear specimens and samples of the resin with entrapped wood chips, pine needles, and insects are easily obtainable at rock shops.

The ancient Chinese believed amber to be the etheric residual left by souls of tigers when they died. The Norse believed that when Freya's tears fell into the sea they became lumps of amber.

This resin exudes a lovely piney scent when burned, and makes a superior disinfectant and fumigant. Since Pliny's time it has enjoyed a reputation as a remedy for ills as varied as toothache, goiter, bladder trouble, heart and lung disease, rheumatism, hysteria, fevers, digestive ailments, headaches, deafness, blindness, and jaundice. Mixed with honey and taken internally, it allegedly quiets coughs and alleviates sore throats.

Cast and break spells with amber. Protect yourself and your children from sorcery by wearing it.

AMETHYST

Rulers: Jupiter, Pisces.

Amethyst is a kind of crystalline quartz colored purple by ferric iron. The quartz forms layers rather like a tree that adds rings every year. Some of the highest quality yet least expensive amethysts are mined in Brazil, where once was discovered a single piece thirty feet long by fifteen yards high that weighed 700 tons. "Saint Valentine Stone" is another name for amethyst, which probably originates in its association with water (= love) signs. In medieval times amethyst was prized more than diamonds. But because it currently floods the market, its value has fallen off. In Greenland, people even use a blue-tinted amethyst to pave paths and driveways!

The stone is alleged to counteract blood disorders, hysteria, gout, insomnia, hallucinations, neuralgia, and anger. An old recipe recommends heating amethyst in water for thirty minutes and using the drops that accumulate on the lid of the pot to erase skin impurities like warts, moles, and freckles.

This stone is associated with the King of Cups in the tarot because it is said to radiate creativity and absolute, yet compassionate power. This is why defendants used to carry the stone into court to influence the outcome of a litigation in their favor. It is also a stone with mystical overtones, and as such, has been fashioned into rings for high officers of the Catholic Church.

Because the stone stands for the high priest, whose mind is not swayed by external phenomena, amethyst is thought to protect against absent-mindedness, blurred thinking, and immoderate drinking. If worn by a Taurus, amethyst will help counteract the negative qualities of this sign. It is also a symbol of philanthropy and friendship. When placed under a pillow, it produces prophetic dreams. Since it falls under the dominion of Pisces, fishermen carry amethyst to secure large catches.

Attach it to wands to invoke spirits. Engrave an amethyst with the signs of the sun and moon, and it will neutralize Black Magic. The versatile amethyst makes an excellent meditation stone that helps a person rise above the troubles of daily life.

AQUAMARINE
Rulers: Uranus, Neptune, Aquarius, Scorpio.

This beryl, whose name means "water from the sea," is usually clear, light green, or blue. It has the same structure as emerald, but is less precious because it is found more commonly in nature.

In times gone by, aquamarine was believed to ameliorate toothache, stress, effects of drug and alcohol abuse, pains in the nerves, neck, jaw, swollen glands, sore throat, and malfunction of the liver, eyes, and stomach.

Under the dominion of Uranus, Neptune, and Aquarius, it is the gem of the mystic, seer, and ocean wanderer. It hones mental vision, and endows the wearer with refined intuition, courage, and a youthful appearance. It restores harmony to family, marriage, and friendships, and brings hope to the oppressed. Aquamarine makes an excellent scrying; that is, divination stone.

Wear aquamarine earrings to attract love. Whenever you are under stress, like during an argument, or before a job interview, hold the stone, and gaze at it for a few minutes. It will help clear your mind and restore your composure.

AVENTURINE

Ruler: Libra.

In its pure form, aventurine is an opaque, greenish quartz with flakes of other colors according to the the minerals in its composition. Hues range from blue and green to red and brown. The stone was once the imperial seal of China and called the "Stone of Heaven."

Gamblers who carry a piece of aventurine in their pockets are said to have the best luck. Keep aventurine on your desk for inspiration when writing.

BLOODSTONE

Ruler: Aries.

Bloodstone, also known as heliotrope or hematite, can be either red or green with blood-red flecks. It is a kind of jasper with the flecks caused by iron oxide.

In the past, people believed that bloodstone stopped bleeding, healed open wounds, acted as a tranquilizer, and aided the digestion.

Bloodstone is used in health spells and rites to bring the possessor a long, happy life. In ancient times in Europe, warriors rubbed powdered bloodstone on their bodies to make themselves invincible. The stone is credited with conferring on the wearer constancy, courage, and endurance. Carrying the stone into court allegedly assures a favorable judgment. Moreover, bloodstone is reputed to stir the passions. It also opens one's paths to the higher.

CARNELIAN

Rulers: Earth, Virgo, Leo.

The ancient name for this stone is "sard," which means "flesh-colored." In actuality, this opaque chalcedony comes in many colors including dark brown, orange, and the popular red. The name in English derives from the Latin word for "flesh," and in the Doctrine of Signatures, stands for carnal passion. In the Bible, carnelian was the first stone on the breastplate of the High Priest of Israel.

Carnelian has long been thought to suppress fears, anger, melancholy, and an overactive imagination. It purifies and rids the blood of poisons and infections, stops the flow of blood, and heals open wounds. It has been used to remedy rheumatism, sore throat, neuralgia, sunstroke, and digestive complaints. Since carnelian allegedly grounds energy, it is ideal for healing.

Wear a carnelian, the symbol of blood ties, to foster love between parent and child. Ancient Greek women used to carry carnelian as a token of chastity. Singers kept it in their pockets to perfect their voices.

Carnelian is considered an effective amulet against accidents, lightning, nightmares, and the evil eye. It is supposed to enable a person to see into the past, although I prefer obsidian for this purpose. As the stone is ruled by Virgo, it stands for family unity and good health. Carnelian enables the possessor to make friends easily, and lifts the spirits.

CHALCEDONY
Rulers: Cancer, Aquarius.

Known as milkstone because of its translucent, whitish-blue color, chalcedony is a type of quartz.

The stone is alleged to absorb poisons and cure fevers, diabetes, and gall stones.

Since chalcedony is said to absorb poison, by analogy, it also neutralizes poisonous thoughts directed at the wearer. In this sense, it deflects negativity and attempts at mind control. It also creates an introspective frame of mind. Chalcedony supposedly attracts good luck, increases physical strength, and improves sour dispositions.

CHRYSOPRASE
Rulers: Moon, Venus, Virgo.

Chrysoprase is an apple-green or golden-colored chalcedony with white streaks. Because of its nickel content, it fades when exposed to light. It is found in Brazil, the Ural Mountains, and the Western United States.

The stone is touted to strengthen the eyesight. Gazing at its calming green color may help balance the personality. In Romanian folklore, the stone is said to enable a person to understand the language of lizards!

Chrysoprase is a protective stone for sea travel, that also eases "cabin fever." Because it is supposed to sharpen physical sight, Witches and Magicians use it to promote fresh insights, attune them to their higher geniuses, and otherwise expand their minds. It is a fine stone to carry when performing a tree meditation, since it is linked with greenery, growth, and new beginnings.

CITRINE
Rulers: Mercury, Gemini, Capricorn.

This yellow or whisky-colored quartz contains iron. It is called "smoky quartz" or "scotch topaz" in Scotland. Artificial citrine is made by heating amethyst to around 900 degrees Fahrenheit, until it turns a golden bronze color.

Many healers believe that smoky quartz locks up psychic energy within its structure. They use the stone in spells that take a long time to bring to fruition, or which require several episodes for completion. Yellow citrine is mined in the Bahian region of Brazil and is called "Bahian Topaz," It is distinguished from genuine topaz mined elsewhere in that country.

By tradition, citrine endows the wearer with the ability to think sensibly about life and remain in control of the emotions. It counterbalances negative thoughts.

CORAL
Rulers: Mars (red), Venus (pink).

Coral is found on the Polynesian reefs. It is organic material built from the calcified skeletons of colonies of tiny sea animals, which is composed of calcium carbonate, magnesium, carbonate, and organic matter. Colors range from orange to pink, red, white, blue and black.

Coral allegedly withstands epidemics. By the Doctrine of Signatures, the red variety is said to staunch the flow of blood and reverse sterility.

By tradition, the stone promotes fertility and sexual attraction, removes curses, brings victory at sea, drives away evil, and protects against violence. This is why some mothers attach it to the bells of their babies' rattles. Ferdinand I of Spain was said to have carried around a piece of coral that he pointed at people when he suspected them of giving him the evil eye.

Coral is an amulet for those who travel by water. It is said that coral grows pale when a loved one is about to die, and conversely, that it darkens when the emotions are stimulated positively.

DIAMOND
Rulers: Saturn, Taurus.

The diamond is the hardest gemstone of all. In fact, in order to cut it, jewelers must use diamond dust. It consists of pure carbon, and is available in a variety of colors from clear (the most common) to black, blue, green, brown, and red.

The best diamonds are found in Africa, although they are obtainable in India, the Urals, Australia, and Brazil, where in recent years large diamond discoveries have been made. Industrial diamonds are easily found, but larger sizes and better quality are rare. The Star of Africa, an enormous stone, weighs over 3,000 carats. Several celebrated cut diamonds have notorious histories, and are supposed to bring bad luck and even death to the possessor.

Diamonds are used to cure maladies of old age such as Alzheimer's disease, hardening of the arteries, and prostate trouble. Elizabeth I of England carried a diamond with her to ward off the plague.

Diamonds symbolize beauty, strength, and power. Those who wish to perfect their inner beings and attain spiritual awareness may wear diamonds as a symbol of their goals. However, the stone can cause the wearer to be jealous and possessive. It tends to magnify both positive and negative personality traits.

In any planetary spell a diamond will help attract and magnify the influence of the required planet. Roman soldiers thought that wearing diamonds next to their bodies emboldened them in battle.

For those of you who wear a diamond on your left hand, you might be interested to know that supposedly you are also protected from wild beasts. Mull that over the next time you're in a singles' bar!

EMERALD
Rulers: Venus, Taurus, Gemini, Libra, Moon, Cancer.

This green beryl, whose color comes from the presence of chromium, occasionally is found in masses as large as pillars. Unfortunately, these large deposits are usually of poor quality.

In ancient Egypt, pregnant women wore the stone around their necks and engraved it with the image of Isis to protect them against miscarriage. The Emerald Tablet of ancient Greek legend, which contained the verses of creation on it, was said to have been written by Hermes, the Mercurian god of wisdom and Magic.

The emerald is a traditional remedy for malaria, nightmares, insomnia, epilepsy, external bleeding, and general bodily weakness. It strengthens the eyesight, intellect, and memory. Emeralds supposedly draw poison from insect bites.

This was the resurrection stone of the ancient Egyptians. Many eyes of Horus were carved from emeralds as a representation of the door to the womb through which the spirit entered to be reborn. Emerald water in homeopathic doses is believed to balance the personality. Emeralds protect the traveller from disaster and enable a person to wax eloquently wherever she/he may journey. The stone is also a marriage talisman and is used in rites of passion and love.

It is reputed to attract psychics and seers to the aura of the wearer, especially when set in gold. It allegedly changes color when a deception against the possessor is afoot. Emeralds bring wisdom and increased cerebral capacities to the wearer.

EYES

Ruler: Sun.

These silky-looking, fibrous quartz pieces are known by various names according to color: cat's eye (olive), tiger's eye (gold), hawk's eye (blue-green). A more expensive cat's eye is chrysoberyl. Eyes include in their composition hornblende, asbestos, phosphorous, and iron.

These stones supposedly cure eye diseases. They also repress asthma attacks, and beautify the skin.

Exotic-looking eyes are ascribed varied magical properties in Voodun. Among them are the powers to arrest the evil eye, control demons, remove spells, help the wearer gain insights into personal faults, and increase psychic potential. Tiger's eye is used in rituals to foster an independent spirit or to promote business interests, and to see into the past and future.

GARNET

Rulers: Mars, Scorpio.

Garnet is a red stone composed of aluminum, calcium, chromium, manganese, and magnesium. Its color is due to the presence of iron.

It also is found in shades of purple, pink, yellow-green, and black. Another name for the stone is "carbuncle." Garnet *en cabochon* refers to a garnet cut with rounded sides.

It is believed that garnets stop hemorrhages and soothe inflammations.

Ruled by Mars, garnet imbues the wearer with the attributes of this fiery planet such as fearlessness, courage, drive, fortitude, good health, and ambition. Garnets also confer a sense of devotion and loyalty. In times gone by, the stone was employed in spells for invisibility and invincibility.

By tradition, wearing a garnet can dissolve a romantic liaison, but on the other hand, it can help find a new lover. In Italy, people call it "the consolation stone" and present it to widows to help them find new mates.

Garnets allegedly possess the power to find hidden treasures and lost objects. Travellers carry garnets for protection, particularly those carved with a lion's head.

JACINTH
Rulers: Aquarius, Uranus (blue), Moon (white), Sagittarius (red).

Also known as zircon, hyacinthe, and the "wishing stone," it is a corundum with a tetragonal shape, and colored yellow, brown, blue, or red. To test its authenticity, subject the stone to heat and it will turn blue. Its appearance is similar to a diamond, but jacinth is doubly refractive, whereas, the diamond is singly refractive.

Stone healers claim they can use jacinth to reduce fever, stimulate digestion, and strengthen the heart.

Jacinth protects travellers and brings them good fortune. It is said that one who wears a jacinth ring is able to peer into the spiritual world and divine the truth, which will appear to the seer in symbolic form. The stone attracts money and power, and helps the wearer avoid natural catastrophes and accidents.

JADE
Rulers: Venus, Moon, Libra.

Jade is called nephrite when composed of calcium, magnesium and iron silicate, and jadeite when consisting of sodium aluminum silicate. The chromium components of some jade create an emerald green color, and the presence of iron is revealed by a bottle-green shade. It is one of the strongest stones that exists, and therefore makes fine weapons and tools.

Jade is alleged to prolong life and protect a person from accidents. Some Mexican and Spanish healers, who call it the "colic stone," administer it in cases of kidney ailments.

Jade has been used for centuries by the Chinese in art and medicine, for they see it as a symbol of the five virtues: mercy, modesty, courage, action, and wisdom. The stone allegedly protects a woman in labor and brings the possessor a large family. Jade restores tranquility, enhances psychic powers, and attracts good fortune. Place jade under your pillow to prevent nightmares. Use it in rituals to seek your internal beauty. Carry it so that your daily life will proceed smoothly and predictably.

JASPER
Rulers: Pluto, Virgo, Libra, Scorpio, Aries.

Jasper is a silicon dioxide found commonly in gravel beds. It is a dark green chalcedony quartz with red flecks caused by the presence of iron oxide. Colors vary from reddish-brown to green and yellow. The red-colored stone is the rarest and most prized. Sometimes it is called heliotrope or bloodstone, and retains some of the same virtues of those stones.

In Iran, doctors powder jasper with turquoise to cure bladder, gall bladder, kidney, and liver complaints. Women who carry jasper or agate with them at the beginning of a pregnancy are supposed to be assured of a safe delivery of a full-term baby. Custom dictates that jasper engraved with a scorpion will improve the sense of smell.

This stone is alleged to kindle the passions, and foster agriculture and horticulture. Some American Indian tribes believed it could make rain. During the waxing moon, place a piece of jasper in a small box with some earth, seal it, and secrete it under your pillow to encourage prophetic dreams. The stone confers courage, wisdom, and constancy in marital relationships. It brings good luck and happiness to the wearer.

LAPIS LAZULI

Rulers: Sun, Jupiter, Taurus.

Called "stone of heaven" by the Egyptians, lapis is made blue by the presence of sulphur. The stone is also faked by dyeing chalcedony blue. You can tell a genuine lapis by the flecks of golden pyrite, although these, too, sometimes can be faked. The Egyptians modelled their scarabs and other jewelry in lapis. They held the stone to be sacred to Isis in her aspect as goddess of truth and justice.

Powdered lapis lazuli makes an ultramarine pigment. The stone enjoys a reputation as a tranquilizer that alleviates painful nerves. It is used by gem healers for diseases of the blood, heart, spleen, and skin, and to calm epileptic fits.

Use lapis in spells to regain love lost, kindle new love and friendship, promote fertility, strengthen the will, protect against evil, and dispel melancholy. The Arabs dedicated this stone to Laz, their love goddess, from whom its name is derived. The Sumerians believed that the person who wore lapis would assimilate the attributes and supernatural powers of the god.

MAGNETITE (LODESTONE)

Ruler: Mars.

Commonly called "lodestone" in magical grimoires, this iron oxide receives its name from the fact that it can be attracted by a magnet.

Because of its magnetizing attributes, the stone can draw shrapnel from wounds. Also it supposedly abates leg cramps, gout pain, fractures, eye and liver ailments, and cures barrenness in women (by attracting a fertile lover?).

Due to its special magnetic properties, magnetite is called the "Hercules stone." Alexander the Great believed so strongly in the powers of this stone that he insisted his soldiers carry small pieces with them as protection from evil spirits. Apply lodestones in charms to draw love (red), prosperity, money, lottery winnings (green), protection, healing (white), and to send back to its source negatively-directed energy (black).

A Voodoo belief recommends carrying magnetite in pairs, as one stone is supposed to ward off negativity, and the other attracts positive vibrations. The wearer can anoint the stone with oil or magnetic sand (iron pyrite, also called "steel dust") depending on the requirements of the spell.

MALACHITE

Rulers: Venus, Aquarius.

Malachite consists of carbonate of copper mixed with water into layers of fine fiber. Its copper content classifies it under the rulership of Venus. It is colored a deep green, and was once called the "peacock stone."

Many medical uses are attributed to malachite. Among them are cures for poisoning, irregular menstruation, toothache, external wounds, colic, cholera, cardiac spasm, eye disorders, and asthma. Egyptian women applied powdered malachite in makeup and hair dye.

By ancient Russian custom, if water is drunk from a cup made of malachite, it enables a person to understand the language of animals. The stone allegedly elevates the spirits, and reinforces the power of spells to influence others. Engraved with the symbol of the sun, it confers omnipotence on the possessor. Given its green color, malachite brings a restful night's sleep to a child if attached to the cradle or bed. Make sure you attach it out of baby's reach: you don't want your child to swallow the stone accidentally!

MOONSTONE

Ruler: Moon.

Common names for this silky stone are "fish eye," "water opal," and "wolf's eye." Like all feldspars, moonstone is composed of aluminum silicate with some potassium. Its glossy, bluish-white luster originates in the potassium and sodium feldspars that separate the stone into thin plates. Moonstones can vary in color from creamy yellow to pink and brown.

This stone is alleged to work successfully in cases of consumption, and female (moon-related) complaints.

Moonstones are the sacred stone of India. They are used in love spells and charms to protect the midnight or water-bound traveller. If you hold a moonstone in your mouth during the full moon, the path to take in the future will become clear. To sew a moonstone into a young woman's clothing is to bless her with many children. Keep a moonstone wrapped in yellow silk to attract prosperity and good luck.

OBSIDIAN

Ruler: Earth.
Obsidian quartz is a black, volcanic lava that was suddenly exposed to air, and solidified so fast it never formed crystals. In other words, it is a natural glass with a smooth surface. Because obsidian is a kind of glass, it is faked by coloring manufactured glass. Color variations include a rainbow sheen, silvery and golden sheen, grayish-white snowflake flecks, and reddish-marbled streaks.

Peering at the shiny surface of a piece of streaked obsidian can bring psychic visions to the trained eye. The Aztecs knew this, and fashioned magic mirrors from polished obsidian. They dedicated the stone to their god, Tezcatlipoca, whose name means "shining mirror." Since psychic vision is sharpened by obsidian, our coven uses it to open the third eye for the "Black Singing Waters" method for past life readings (see *Web of Light*, pp. 176-179).

ONYX

Rulers: Saturn, Capricorn.
Another black stone, onyx is a banded chalcedony. Artisans carve it into items such as ashtrays, bookends, statues, and chess sets. Also known as "black amber," the lovely snowflake onyx is sprinkled with delicate white flecks that form snowflake patterns. Brazilian, or Mexican onyx is another stone, a banded calcite. Some unscrupulous dealers will sell black glass for onyx —— so beware!

The stone improves hearing and ear troubles. By analogy, it hones listening skills. Homeopathic doses are said to be inspirational. Onyx supposedly cures heart and circulatory disorders, and soothes watery eyes. It strengthens and beautifies the hair, nails, and skin.

In Elizabethan times, Magicians made magic mirrors from onyx. As a black stone it is associated with darkness and is carried to ward off the evil eye and keep rivals away from a spouse or suitor. It allegedly chases away nightmares. Choose onyx to meditate on matters that require a good deal of concentration or inspiration. For this reason, many rosaries are made from onyx beads.

A gift of onyx to a newborn reputedly insures that the child will be able to settle all debts within the first thirty years of life. Onyx brings tranquility and courage in the face of danger. In another tradition which equates the color black with evil, it rains misfortune and destroys marriages.

OPAL

Rulers: Mercury, Moon, Neptune, Scorpio, Pisces, Uranus (fire opal).

Opal is a silica filled with air and water that changes its molecular structure from a hexagonal to a grape-like formation. The percentage of water can vary from six to thirty-four percent of the weight of the stone, and often minute cracks appear due to the action of the water. Do not expose it to light for prolonged periods or it may dry out and become dull. To preserve your opal keep it in water or oil.

The water content of this quartz makes it iridescent. Colors can vary from milky white to green, yellow, and dark red. Do not let a seller take these stones outside in daylight to show them off because the bright light makes them appear more attractive than they really are.

Opals have acquired the reputation of improving the eyesight and memory, and retaining the blond hair color of the light-haired wearer. Gem healers believe that since the stone "vibrates" on an intensely high energy level, it should not be worn by anyone with a nervous disorder.

The name of this gem comes from a Sanskrit term meaning "valuable stone." The ancient Greeks and Romans thought the opal could reveal the future to its owner; so they called it the "gem of the gods." When life went well for the possessor, it reputedly sparkled brilliantly; when circumstances were about to take a bad turn, the stone darkened.

Opal allegedly awakens the sensual nature. It is employed in invisibility spells, and spells to contact the spirit world.

However, the stone claims an unfortunate reputation for the royal families of England, Spain, and Sweden. It is also considered a bad luck stone, and the stone of thieves in Russian tradition. Perhaps because of this association, opals are exploited in Black Magic as cursing weapons.

PEARL

Rulers: Cancer, Moon.

Deep inside the oyster or mussel where a grain of sand or other impurity lodges, the magnificent natural pearl is born. The mollusk excretes layer upon layer of calcium carbonate to coat the irritation, which eventually forms a pearl. Because of their maritime origin, pearls were once called "stones of the sea."

The pearl's specific lustrous color depends on the temperature of the water in which it is discovered. Pink-tinted pearls are found off the coast of Sri Lanka, cream, on the Persian Gulf, green in Japan, blue near Australia, and brown and black in the Gulf of Mexico. Regrettably, pearls lose their luminescence over time, especially when exposed to light. Nevertheless, they are an elegantly understated precious stone, ultra feminine in their softness, and much desired by women.

For what it's worth, in a television interview I saw in the U.K. the former British Prime Minister, Margaret Thatcher, remarked that the pearl is her personal favorite jewel and that she believes it is the one stone that shows the English feminine skin to its best advantage! In folklore it is claimed that pearls improve the quality and tone of the skin.

The ancients believed that pearls helped alleviate the stomach discomfort of ulcers, regulate the female menstrual cycle, and cure fevers. The Mogul emperors used to drink decoctions of pearls to increase their virility. The Chinese thought that cloud dragons rained "pearl drops" from the sky that were gobbled up by oysters and retained in their shells. This precious bodily fluid of the gods was alleged to cure a range of diseases from near-sightedness to plague.

The pearl's unfortunate reputation is linked to greed, cruelty, and suffering. Often it is likened to a teardrop, an allusion to the sorrow that it is suspected of visiting upon its owner. On the positive side, pearls are linked to purity, and are alleged to calm the savage breast.

An interesting description of the fascinating history of pearls occurs in the mystery novel, *Pearlhanger*, by Jonathan Gash. Lovejoy, antiques dealer extraordinaire, relates:

> "Funny thing, but some gems — and the pearl is a classified gemstone, remember — are special. They appeal to something in the mind. The pearl is one. Passion and igno- rance have haunted it. Like, the Incas of Peru used to cook

oysters just to extract the pearl. I ask you. And Sir Thomas Gresham drank Queen Bess's health in wine containing pearl powder made by grinding up a huge and precious pearl. Well, Sir Thomas was only doing what Cleopatra and Claudius the famous Roman glutton used to do....You see how romance and pearls go together? But it's often romance of a peculiar and oddly rather sinister kind. Like, you can't call Caligula's huge pearl necklace romantic, because it was named for his favorite horse. And his wife Lollia Paulina's craving for pearls was too passionate for sanity, though that was par for the course in Caligula's household. They were all loony.

"Men wore them too, hung as a little clapper in a tiny gold bell earring. It became such a craze that Caesar put a stop to these *crotalia*, little rattles, because unmarried women were wearing them as a sexy invitation. Some say that Julius Caesar invaded (Britain) simply to capture the Old World's best source of freshwater pearls."[10]

PERIDOT

Ruler: Libra.

Peridot is a kind of agate formerly known as green chrysolite. Another name for it is "olivine."

The stone allegedly heals gout. According to gem healers, it also displays the usual qualities associated with other green stones.

Peridot helps a person perform research more easily, and attain wisdom. By tradition, it bestows innocent pleasures, and enjoyment of the simple, modest things of life.

Peridot was a favorite stone of the ancient Roman soldiers, who carried it with them to faraway lands to allay pangs of homesickness, delusions, and fears. It is considered a marriage stone for those who would hasten into matrimony. It neutralizes the negative effects of female betrayal, attracts friends, and energizes the body.

QUARTZ CRYSTAL

Rulers: Leo (gold), Gemini (clear), Capricorn (smoky).

Quartz combines silicon and oxygen into hexagonal crystals interspersed with blank spaces. If the blank spaces are filled by minerals, the quartz becomes colored. Examples of colored quartz include citrine (iron), aventurine (mica flakes), smoky (aluminum), rose (titanium, manganese), amethyst (ferric iron). Quartz forms twelve per cent of the earth's crust.

Agate, bloodstone, carnelian, chalcedony, chrysoprase, jasper, and onyx all possess crystalline structures, but so small as to appear to lack any structure at all. Opal is a silica gel without the crystal form into which water has been mixed. Silky tiger's eye has fibrous inclusions of iron silicate.

In industry, mostly human-made quartz crystals are employed in computers, transistors, and laser technology. In times past, quartz was considered a healing stone of such high repute that it was sold in pharmacies as late as the middle of the eighteenth century. Allegedly quartz stops the flow of blood and diarrhea, encourages new mothers to produce milk, and alleviates sunburn, vertigo, and anxiety.

Formerly quartz was thought to be frozen water; so the ancients placed it in fields to attract rain. By the same reasoning, the Chinese put a small crystal on their tongues to suppress thirst when travelling across the desert. Inca and North American Indians buried their dead with a piece of crystal because they believed the stone contained a spark of divinity that would draw the soul on its journey toward the light. Early Christians saw in quartz a symbol of the immaculate conception. Other cultures believed that the stone could render opaque objects invisible.

The belief in quartz as a healing stone originates in its alleged power to capture and imprison illness inside the voids between its crystals. The more a quartz crystal is used for healing purposes, so the story goes, the more energy it acquires. One famous Irish crystal has seemed to cure cattle of disease for centuries. Farmers place it in a running stream and drive their cattle through the water. The powers of this crystal are reputed to have increased over time.

If you apply quartz for healing, gem healers suggest you recharge the crystal with the specific energy you require each time you use it. To drain it completely of energy, they recommend using magnetite.

Of course, it is a well-known fact that neither quartz crystals nor any other stone can physically conduct an electrical charge in measurable terms. What I refer to here is a psychic charge, immeasurable by current scientific tools. The psychic charge held by a crystal may not even be similar to a physical electrical charge. However, since this is what it (as well as many other psychic manifestations) feels like, we have no other adequate vocabulary with which to describe it. Someday we may be able to measure these phenomena with scientific accuracy, and perhaps then we will find an appropriate language to describe them. Until that time, we must suffer the misinformation disseminated by the credulous, superstitious, and untrained, as well as the derision of the narrow-minded scientific community whose world view is too structured to understand the symbolic language through which by necessity we communicate.

Quartz is considered an important scrying tool, perhaps because of the intricate play of light that dances and shimmers off the surfaces and fires the imagination. Crystal gazers often speak of what appears to be a vibration that occurs after they gaze for some time at a crystal. The effect on the brain is so convincing that they swear it can be discerned by other perceptive eyes. Quartz points also make fine pendulums.

Quartz is a power stone that enables Witches to persuade others to do their bidding. It is also a key component in rainmaking spells.

ROSE QUARTZ
Rulers: Venus, third decanate of Virgo, Libra, Taurus.

A beautifully refined colored stone that receives its blushing hue from manganese, rose quartz unfortunately is solar-sensitive and can lose its color when overexposed to sunlight. When you choose a piece of rose quartz, verify that the color is distributed evenly.

This gentle stone evokes young artists, poets, sculptors, mediums, and all people who are sensitive and delicate. Rose quartz is alleged to calm passions. It makes a fine gift for a girl on her first communion, or on graduating from high school.

RUBY
Rulers: Mars, Aries.

Ruby is a corundum that crystallizes in a trigonal system. Colored red from aluminum, carat for carat, rubies are even more precious than diamonds. Perhaps this is why the Hindus call it the "king of precious stones." Another name for this gem is "carbuncle," although some cuts of garnets also are called by that name.

Because rubies are red, Sympathetic Magic dictates that they be used to strengthen the heart and purify the air. Rubies are a traditional cure for fevers, plague, internal pains, and the discomfort of miscarriage. They also supposedly prevent tooth decay.

The ruby's red color radiates strength and protection and therefore, stands for justice. The stone is a logical choice for charms for psychic self-defense because it helps spur action, and reputedly arouses creative, energetic, independent thought.

As the story goes, the ruby now ensconced in the Imperial State Crown of the English Crown Jewels originally was mounted in the coronet of King Henry V's helmet, which he wore into the Battle of Agincourt. The enemy smote the king with a sword, but only was able to break off part of the coronet on the helmet— the part that held the ruby.

Rubies chase away sad thoughts and motivate procrastinators. This versatile stone may help you act on the courage of your convictions. It symbolizes passionate love, yet on a more spiritual plane than jasper. The ruby makes an excellent pommel stone for magical tools, and is reported to enhance the wearer's powers of intuition. Finally, it enjoys a reputation as an aphrodisiac!

SAPPHIRE
Rulers: Jupiter, Saturn (the name in Greek means "beloved of Saturn"), Virgo, Gemini (yellow), Taurus (blue), Aquarius.

Sapphire is a hard corundum which can vary in color from white to yellow, bluish-green, light blue, and dark blue, the azure color being the most coveted. The stone is found in Burma, Ceylon, the Arab Emirites, Sri Lanka, New South Wales, and Persia. Some also are mined in Montana. To date, the largest sapphire discovered weighed 950 carats. When light shines on sapphire it is deflected into the shape of a pentagram. For this reason the stone is prized by Witches, who consider the pentagram their emblem.

The stone allegedly counterbalances melancholy and insomnia, and is a remedy for nervous disorders, madness, eye troubles, fever, asthma, blood efusions such as nosebleed, and is a poison antidote. Star sapphires help cure ulcers and eye diseases. Sky-blue sapphire is considered male, and and carries a strong healing capacity. The female sea-blue sapphire assuages ulcers and nosebleeds.

In the Buddhist faith, sapphires represent devotion and spiritual enlightenment. Gem healers believe the stone repairs the nervous system and infuses a person with the joy and innocence of youth. This versatile gem helps the wearer develop true friendship and love, and induces peace of mind. It is an effective defense against false friends and Black Magic. Traditionally, sapphires are worn by yogis, healers, and saints because they confer clear vision and insight. The star sapphire protects from evil and attracts good fortune and love.

SARDONYX

Ruler: Virgo.

Sardonyx is a type of layered chalcedony that combines reddish-brown chalcedony (formerly called "sard") with black and white layers. It is a favorite stone for carving cameos and intaglios. Medicinally, it is touted to neutralize poisons from bites and all infections.

The stone attracts new friends, marital happiness and success of the type that often leads to high position and monetary gain. Gazing at it is said to stimulate the mind. In ancient Greece, lawyers carried the stone into court to aid eloquence. Traditionally, it is an amulet against sorcery.

SERPENTINE

Rulers: Scorpio, Cancer.

The name signifies "snakelike stone," and was so called because of its markings that resemble those of a viper. Serpentine is a green stone, but also is found in black and white shades. It is fibrous in nature, and contains other minerals such as asbestos and chrysolite. Serpentine feels oily to the touch, like soapstone.

Serpentine protects against poison and venomous animals.

TOPAZ

Rulers: Sun, Sagittarius.

Topaz is a corundum made from aluminum hydroxyl flourine silicate. Its colors vary from red to blue, green, colorless, and yellow, the yellowish-gold hue being the most common. Its crystal forms an irregular rhombic shape. The finest topazes are mined in Minas Gerais and Rio Grande do Sul in Brazil. Beware of the so-called Bahian (Brazilian) topaz, as it is actually citrine, a yellow quartz.

The stone is supposed to heal circulatory problems, varicose veins, thrombosis, piles, hemorrhage, liver complaints, rheumatism, and insomnia. In times past, it was considered an antidote to insanity.

The golden-colored topaz receives its color from phosphorous, which becomes brighter or duller according to the waxing or waning moon. Thus the powers of the gold topaz ebb and flow with moon phases.

The gem is named after a legendary island in the Red Sea that means "to seek." Keywords associated with this stone are: nobility, courage, leadership, wisdom, and regal splendor. The stone allegedly changes color near poison. Topaz furthers friendships, builds trust, destroys the evil eye, and helps eliminate fear of death. It also defends against vengeful enemies. A gift of topaz (as in my opinion, any gem) brings happiness to the wearer.

The gold-colored topaz is associated with the solar power of the animal kingdom of which the lion is the king. In human terms, this is translated into a symbol of the transformation of lower animal passions and baser natures into that which is pure and noble.

Topaz is alleged to help find buried treasure, but in my opinion, if you own a topaz, you already possess a treasure.

TOURMALINE
Rulers: Sun, Mercury, Gemini.

Tourmaline occurs in different colors, but it is bicolored with one half clear green and the other half, pink. Black tourmaline is called "Brazilian sapphire." When this gem flecks quartz with what looks like penetrating black rays, the quartz is known as "tourmalated quartz." Other colors include blue, yellow, brown, and red. Tourmaline is a complex stone with twenty different constituents including quartz, feldspar, mica, hornblende, and iron.

In Sri Lanka, men rub it in wool until it becomes charged with static electricity in order to clean tobacco ash from their pipes because warmed tourmaline attracts small particles from the air. Tourmaline is attributed with the power to cure plague, consumption, infections, and blood poisoning. Reputedly it arrests decomposition in dead bodies.

The stone is a token of friendship and good will. It symbolizes the joy of living, and imbues the wearer with greater self-confidence and inner radiance. The stone is highly recommended for meditation, especially the soothing, clear blue and green colors. It is considered as a lucky charm for those involved in the performing arts, writers, and artists.

TURQUOISE
Rulers: Sun, Venus (sky-blue), Saturn (ice-blue), Uranus, Aquarius (green-blue) Capricorn, Earth.

Turquoise is composed of silica, ammonia, water, and copper and aluminum phosphates. It is a granular, fibrous, opaque stone of great beauty, used for jewelry and decoration by Egyptians and American Indians. The color can vary from green (predominance of ferric iron) to sky-blue (predominance of copper). It is a sensitive stone that will fade unless it is kept safe from sun and heat, soap, perfume, and perspiration.

It's name means "Turkish stone," as the Turks believed it to be a lucky gem. Turquoise allegedly cures heart trouble and malaria.

The color is supposed to fade when its owner feels ill or threatened. Because it absorbs negative influences, it makes a superior protective stone, particularly for children. It is a prized gift bestowed by American Indians on newborns. Curiously, turquoise raised similar associations in the minds of the Egyptians, who linked the stone with Hathor, the mother goddess. It also withstands melancholy, and brings peace to domestic disputes.

Turquoise was sacred to the Persians, who believed that its sky-blue color symbolized true love and innocence. An old superstition claims that turquoise should be given, not bought for yourself. Its color is conducive to meditation.

To make a wish come true, on the hour and day of Jupiter, hold the stone in your right hand and say your wish aloud. Concentrate on the power penetrating your hand, and spreading throughout your body. When you feel the power reach your heart, your wish will be granted.

According to legend, turquoise relieves marital tension, protects horses, and prevents spills from horses. Place turquoise outside on the night of the new moon, and in the morning, bring it in, place it in a charm bag, and carry it with you. You will receive fortunate news!

Chapter 5:
Talismans

A rabbit's foot in your pocket, dice jingling from the car's rear view mirror, a class ring on your finger - whether we realize it or not, we all encounter, and perhaps however unconsciously, rely on talismans in our daily lives.

A talisman is an inanimate object charged with a particular force that is believed to enable the person for whom it is intended to achieve a preconceived aim by attracting the force with which it is charged from the energy pool of the universe. Usually it is carried in pocket or purse, or attached to the wearer's clothing so that its power to attract is always at hand. A talisman reinforces the will of the person carrying it, and in this sense, acts like a sword (in some magical systems, the symbol of the Magician's will).

A related kind of magical object is known as an amulet. Statues of saints, Christian crosses, Egyptian eyes of Horus and the like, by tradition, are considered to possess the ability to protect people from bad luck and other malefic influences. Belief in amulets originated with the ancient concept of fetishes, which are objects that were thought to house a special spirit or genie. Amulets protect, and in this way, are worn like a shield.

Since some things that contain supposed intrinsic amuletory powers also are charged by Witches and Magicians for other specific purposes, confusion can arise when identifying talismans and amulets, and the terms often are used interchangeably. This chapter is concerned primarily with talismans in the classic meaning of the word.

What items people choose, why they carry talismans, and how talismans work, is something of a mystery. From an etymological point of view this is appropriate, since the name derives from an Arabic word, *tilsam,* meaning "mystery."

People tend to select talismans on the basis of their personal values. An object's age, its geographical origin, the value of the material from which it is made, and the universality of its symbolic meaning or inscription, all help determine what a person will choose as a talisman. This is why ancient Indian arrowheads, small stones from the vicinity of the pyramids at Karnac, gemstones, and articles carved with sacred figures such as pentagrams, hexagrams, eyes of Horus, and runic signs have become popular lucky charms.

The reason why people value them is more difficult to understand. Undeniably, people from all cultures at every time in history have esteemed talismans, but what civilizations consider talismanic depends on their values, attitudes, customs, and beliefs. Some symbols strike a universal chord while others remain quite personal, valued only by the individual.

The Doctrine of Signatures, which dates back to the time of Paracelsus, may form a basis for the belief in talismans. This theory posits that "like produces like" and also that once two things have come into contact, they continue to influence each other mutually by magical means.

C.G. Jung called this phenomenon "synchronicity," and used it to account for why some people are lucky, and others seem unlucky, or how people have runs of good and bad luck. According to Jung, a certain relationship exists between a person's psychological state and the events that are attracted to this person. The link, however, is subtle, and difficult to define. Certainly, it is not as simple as the advocates of the power of positive thinking say when they exhort people to change their behavior patterns. If they think happy, positive thoughts, these optimists claim, all will turn out for the best.

Certainly, belief plays a large part in how talismans function in much the same way as faith healing. People's perceptions of good and bad luck differ widely from culture to culture, and even from individual to individual. Nonetheless, there seems to be more than meets the eye to the punch that talismans pack.

In Magic we attempt to reinforce some synchronic links in order to work toward the betterment of the individual and society. Some Occultists believe that the charm itself is of little value, but that once consecrated and charged with a particular force, it continues to draw similar energy from the universe, and will fulfill its appointed purpose unless the energy current is willfully interrupted.

The theory behind the inner workings of Talismanic Magic is related to how all Magic functions, and is a complex subject, which I discuss in *Secrets of a Witch's Coven*. Suffice it to say that it takes dedication to the study of the principles of Magic and steady practice to become adept at charging talismans. A joke circulating among Occultist groups is that anyone who can effectively charge a talisman really does not need one.

Notwithstanding, I find that some talismans can be charged successfully by people with some basic knowledge of the Craft who follow appropriate procedures. Later in this book I will give you a talisman consecration ritual.

Discussion of some objects that have served as common talismans throughout the ages follows. These items include tools, representations of body parts and articles of clothing, plants and animals, inscriptive talismans, and Egyptian charms. Sacred stones and gems, which were dealt with in chapter 4, also constitute valuable talismans.

In the descriptions that follow, I note if the object has any significance in tea leaf reading, since divination by tea leaves is also addressed in this book.

Tools

Because they were instrumental to people's survival, from earliest times tools were ascribed extraordinary powers. Often they were carved with the name of the person who wore them or the force they typified. Some tools, such as the dagger and sword, were elevated to the stature of ritual weapons, and used for religious and magical purposes.

ARROW

Tea leaves: bad news.

Because arrows swiftly and competently killed game and tribal enemies, they were accredited with miraculous powers. In many ancient cultures, arrows represent sun power, and are depicted in paintings as sunrays streaming from a solar disc. The arrow also reminds us of virility and desire, as in Cupid's piercing love arrows. In runecasting, the Nordic rune in the shape of an arrow means victory in accordance with divine law, plots, gossip, or secret romance.

AX

Tea leaves: troubles, difficulties are overcome.

Even in Neolithic times, this tool, with its clean cutting edge, fundamental for the creation of heat and shelter, was thought to symbolize the divine being. Civilizations as diverse as Celts and Japanese wove myths around the origin of this sacred weapon. The Celts thought the fairies introduced this weapon to mortals, while the Japanese believed that the first ax was dropped from the sky by spirits flying overhead.

CHAIN

Tea leaves: trouble ahead; constriction of independence.

While chains can bind in a negative sense, they also can link or unite in a positive way. Thus, the sign also stands for union, agreement, bonding, successful communication, and marriage.

FAN

Tea leaves: flirtation; discretion advised.

In Western mythology, fans typify the lunar power of flux and reflux. Since the moon is associated with sex from a feminine perspective, an entire fan language has developed around the concept of the fan as it relates to the hidden meanings of female eroticism. This is how the divinatory meaning of the word originated. Probably the Spaniards are best known for elevating this mode of secret sexual communication to an art form.

In Oriental cultures, fans show the power of air, and a person's high rank.

HAMMER
Tea leaves: triumph over adversity; ruthlessness; headaches in the workplace.

Nordic myth has it that the hammer possesses the mystic power of creation. The Norse thought that if they wore this emblem around their necks they would draw the protection of the all-powerful god, Thor, whose symbol is the hammer, and that warriors would thereby gain ferociousness and courage in battle.

KNIFE
Tea leaves: quarrels; separation with ill feeling; near the handle of the cup, divorce.

Besides symbolizing the Witch's will in the form of the magical dagger, called the Athame, knives in general represent death, sacrifice, and vengeance. If elongated into a sword, the meaning changes to the triumph of the spirit over adverse circumstances. In Jungian symbology, the knife represents the shadow self.

LADDER
A ladder pictured in a tea cup signifies advancement through hard work, or indicates that conditions will improve.

SCISSORS
Tea leaves: fights; separation; near the handle, domestic strife.

This ambivalent symbol represents both birth and death, creation and destruction. In mythology, scissors were used by the mystic spinners who cut the thread of life.

WAGON
When pictured in a tea cup, a wagon shows a rough journey, either on the physical or mental plane. Ironically, a wagon can also stand for a wedding.

WHEEL
Tea leaves: advancement through personal effort, good fortune, a positive destiny.

The wheel is an ancient symbol of the power of the sun and the effects of the cosmic tides within the passage of time; hence the term, Great Wheel of Life. It also signifies spiritual illumination.

Body Parts and Articles of Clothing

The human body and what we use to cover our nakedness have proven fertile ground for talismans and amulets in all civilizations.

EYE
Tea leaves: caution; take heed; someone is watching the inquirer.
Known to the ancient Egyptians as the *udjat*, "eye of Horus," or "eye of the Sun God," it was painted on the incisions made in mummies in order to protect and keep them healthy in the afterlife. People wore jewelry fashioned into eyes to shield them from the malicious glances of jealous rivals, and to provide them with the bounty of the sun.

HAT
Tea leaves: repression; a secret marriage; a new job; diplomacy; at the bottom of the cup, a rival.
Because hats are used to cover the head, the crown of one's being, to wear a hat shows a desire to conceal one's true identity, and become what one is not, or what one would like to be. Hence, the expression "to wear many hats." Masks express similar connotations. The hat also is viewed as a kind of badge of office that symbolizes a person's authority in a certain field, such as a hardhat for a construction worker, a policeman's cap, a monarch's crown, or a graduate's mortar board.

HAND
Tea leaves: strength; friendship; charity; union; facing upward, a plea for help.
Images of the human hand held in different positions have epitomized many concepts in different cultures. One of the most renowned is the outstretched hand of Fatima, an Arabic talisman usually struck in metal. It typifies the Moslem holy family, with the

thumb representing the Prophet, and the fingers his four companions. The five commandments of their sect, for which the hand serves as a reminder, are: keep the Feast of Ramadan, accomplish a pilgrimage to Mecca, give alms, perform the necessary ablutions and oppose all infidels. An image of a hand with a pine cone on the thumb and a snake curved around the ring finger is alleged to increase the potency of the charm.

In Brazil, the hand held in a fist with the thumb protruding from between the first and second fingers is a potent protective force that makes the wearer invulnerable to misfortune. A large *figa* (as it is called) is placed in the bedroom facing the door so no evil may enter. However, in tea leaf reading, a clenched fist means a quarrel.

HEART
Tea leaves: love; when broken, unlucky in love; with an arrow pointing downward, someone will harm you; with an arrow pointing upward, someone will protect you; with an arrow straight across, someone is smitten with you.

The heart embodies the life force of the individual. In Egypt, the *ab*, as it was named, comprised the seat of the soul, and was imagined to contain the soul of Khepera, the self- created, self-existing god. It symbolizes the power of the unconscious mind as well as eternity, and is an apt talisman for development of psychic potential. The heart also symbolizes our secret centers and the seat of human valor.

SHOE
According to traditional tea leaf reading, shoes suggest both liberty and the female sex organ. A shoe pictured in a cup indicates that delayed news will be positive.

UMBRELLA
Tea leaves: protection; mourning; troubles; if the umbrella is closed, no shelter will be found.

The general symbolism of the umbrella is two-fold: on one hand, it represents shade from the searing sun; on the other, its phallic shape suggests paternal figures.

Flora and Fauna

Ever observant about the natural world, and drawing correspondences between nature and human life, our forefathers educed numerous talismanic meanings from flora and fauna. Often they carried on their bodies or in their clothes images of these things so that they might acquire their virtues. In other books, I deal with the symbolism of some animals, trees, flowers, and other plants. Here I give you a small sampling of the more ubiquitous symbols.

ACORN
Tea leaves: progress, savings; near the middle of the side of the cup, better health; near the top, financial success.

Among the many fruits and berries sacred to the Celts and Druids, the acorn was chosen to characterize the blessings of the Lord and Lady. A meal ground from these nuts saw people through the long, hard winters; thus the acorn was considered a sustainer of life.

Since its shape resembles the male sex organ, it also became a charm for virility and fertility. Carrying a dried acorn allegedly helps the wearer maintain a youthful appearance.

APPLE
Tea leaves: thirst for knowledge; a long life; achievement.

Because of its spherical shape, the apple symbolizes totality. The fruit also reflects physical desire; hence the meaning of the apple in the Garden of Eden.

EGG
Tea leaves: positive changes; success; fertility.

In many cultures, the egg epitomizes immortality and the ineffable mystery of life. The Egyptians proclaimed it a symbol of the afterlife. Alchemists believed that the egg was the receptacle for matter and thought. In Protective Magic eggs guard against the evil eye. In some primitive cultures, eggs were used as a cure for sterility.

FLOWER
Tea leaves: your wish will be granted.

Because flowers are beautiful, but of a transitory nature, they are linked with beauty and springtime. Since the shape of many flowers resembles a solar disc radiating from a central point, this center is considered representative of the soul. The interpretation of an individual flower depends on many factors, including color, size, shape, and fragrance. (See *Witch's Brew* for a detailed description of flowers and their significance.)

FOUR-LEAFED CLOVER
Tea leaves: good luck, prosperity; inquirer may have more than one lover.
A well-known Irish charm, so goes the folksaying about the four-leafed clover: one leaf is for fame, another for wealth, yet a third for a faithful lover, and the last for glorious health.

LEAF
Tea leaves: good news, fulfillment of ambitions; leaves in a cluster, happiness.
In Chinese tradition, a leaf symbolizes happiness. Several leaves in a bunch stand for people, or humanity in general. The kind of tree the leaf is from also holds important symbolic value. I discuss the meanings of trees at length in *Web of Light*.

LOTUS
The elegant lotus hails from the Orient, where because of its pure, delicate flower, born from the muddy waters, yet not defiled by them, it was judged to be of superhuman origin. The flower means good luck, wealth, fortune, and beauty. In Egypt, this "lily of the celestial ocean" stood for fertility and fruitfulness. The emblem was adopted by Qabalists, and more recently, incorporated into David Palladini's Aquarian tarot deck.

MUSHROOM
Tea leaf reading: expansion.
If the image appears near the cup handle, the inquirer will make a new home abroad. Mushrooms also signify the bounty of the earth. In a negative sense, they can refer to a situation that has ranged out of control.

PALM TREE
Tea leaves: a trip to a faraway land; money; the good life; victory.

Palm trees represent fertility. In Jungian terms, they depict the *anima*.

PINE CONE
Tea leaves: strength

A Semitic symbol of fertility and long life, the pine cone also is related to the Greek goddess, Cybele, and her power and prosperity. In times gone by, people skewered pine cones on poles and staked them in vineyards in the belief that they protected tender grapes from blight and other calamaties.

SHELL
Tea leaves: love; a happy, comfortable life in the next world.

Due to its maritime origin, the sea shell is an image of fertility and femininity. In Chinese tradition, shells confer good luck and prosperous journeys.

BAT
Tea leaves: a false friend, plots against the inquirer; protection.

Unfortunately, bats have received a lot of bad press from Western traditions based on the misconceived notion that they are demons that feed on human blood. Maybe they earned this reputation because they "hang around" caves, cemeteries, barns, and other forlorn places. So in folklore, to hear a bat cry or to encounter a bat harbingers ill luck.

On the other hand, the Chinese believe that the nocturnal creature bestows long life and happiness.

BEAR
Tea leaves: obstacles; danger as the result of a bad decision; an awkward person; if the figure is turned away from the handle, a long trip.

In the symbology of psychology, bears typify our perilous inner thoughts, instincts, and the unconscious mind. On the other hand, the fact that bears hibernate in the winter and emerge from their lairs in the spring, symbolizes rebirth.

In Appalachia, a gift to a baby of bear teeth is said to strengthen the baby's teeth.

BEE

Tea leaves: domestic bliss; good news; a busy time; monetary gain; near the handle, a successful gathering; a swarm of bees, public success.

Different cultures throughout the ages have sought in the industrious bee a reminder of the virtues of diligence, hard work, and obedience, which produce creativity and wealth. In ancient Egypt, the bee was honored as a symbol of royalty.

To bring success to your business, have your bee talisman cast in silver or gold. According to superstition, if you find a bee trapped in your house you are in for a spell of good luck.

BIRD

Tea leaves: if in flight, a message of good news; leadership; if at rest, a happy trip; family.

Birds remind us of the lofty heights of the spiritual plane, the soul, and by analogy, the sun and storms. The great store set by birds in many civilizations probably stems from their unpredictable, but seemingly purposeful flight patterns. The Garuda, an East Indian bird, is accredited with protecting the home and its inhabitants. In Scandinavian myth, an enormous bird is held responsible for creating the world by beating its enormous wings.

BULL

Tea leaves: creativity; fertility; strength; an enemy; quarrels; stubbornness.

The bull carries both lunar/female and solar/male connotations. In the most ancient religious cults, this animal was esteemed as representative of the Earth Mother, the projection of the fecund female principle. As solar cults came to predominate, the concept of the will was depicted by the bull, who penetrates the female principle with its masculinity. It also signified the superiority of mammals over reptiles.

BUTTERFLY

Tea leaves: silly but enjoyable pastimes; scattered thoughts; if surrounded by dots, the inquirer will spend money on frivolous things.

This lovely creature is a Gnostic talisman for resurrection and rebirth. I have seen it etched into Welsh love spoons (talismanic spoons carved from a single piece of wood, and displayed in homes), where it refers to domestic harmony and bliss.

COW
The prosaic cow nonetheless provides milk and meat to human life. To the Egyptians, this important symbol illustrated the potency of Hathor, ruler of childbirth, beauty, and creation. She always appears as a cow-headed deity.

DOG
Tea leaves: a faithful friend.
As in the tea leaf message, dogs symbolize faithfulness and also protection, as well as the Guiding Light. At one time dogs were believed to be companions of the dead. A dog howling at the full Moon is said to presage death.

DRAGON
Tea leaves: obstacles, great power; a sudden change.
Resembling, but not actually a part of the natural world, the mythological dragon possesses talismanic attributes in several cultures, and in some like the Chinese, Tibetan, and Welsh, was elevated to the status of an emblematic figure. This imposing creature is accredited with bringing good fortune, luck, material gain, longevity, and domestic bliss in Oriental and Welsh symbology.

EAGLE
Tea leaves: favorable news; power and fame.
The mighty bird, admired for its size, capacity for survival in the high places of the world, independence, keen eye, and devastating claw, is the emblem of the United States of America. Because the eagle also denotes longevity, many American Indians thought that eagle feathers would somehow consume other feathers if they were laid together in a pile. As a talisman, the figure confers heightened perception, dignity, and favorable treatment by the powers that be.

FISH

Tea leaves: salvation; the inquirer will lead a charmed life; invitation to a meal; several fish, disappointment.

The fish that nowadays is associated with Christianity, is highly significant in many religions. The Hindus proclaim it is the incarnation of Vishnu, and represents fertility and prosperity. The cow-headed goddess, Hathor, whom you met above, also was linked with fish in the minds of the Egyptians. The fish became an Egyptian talisman for prosperity, abundance, fertility, and marital happiness. It is alleged that if you cast your fish talisman in gold or mother of pearl, it will bless you with a large family.

HEN

In tea leaf reading the materialization of a hen presages a birth in the family and domestic bliss.

HORSE

Tea leaves: by tradition, a horse's head means the appearance of a lover; a galloping horse brings good news.

Horses hold different significances for various cultures. They can personify both fire and light, and sometimes are taken to foreshadow death and destruction, as in the Four Horsemen of the Apocalypse.

In Celtic lands, to dream of a white horse means death is imminent. However, if a pair of lovers sees a white horse, blessings are in store. Other cultures have discerned in the horse a symbol of our most potent instincts and desires. Superstition dictates that piebald horses are portents of good luck. A British superstition claims that to insert horsehairs into a child's sandwich will cure the child of worms.

LION

Tea leaves: the inquirer will conquer all enemies and be prosperous, perhaps with the help of an influential friend.

Long perceived as a symbol of the regenerative powers of the sun, the king of beasts presided over the annual fertilizing flood in ancient Egypt. The life-giving flood occurred when the sun passed through the zodiac sign, Leo the Lion. In Greece, along with the bull, the lion characterized the sun-god, Mithras.

MONKEY
Tea leaves: self-deception, dangerous flattery.

In Chinese mythology, the monkey is like the Occidental notion of elemental spirits and fairies. These spirits confer health, wealth, success, and protection. On the other hand, in Western symbology, the monkey incarnates the baser instincts of our unconscious minds — probably because many Westerners regard this animal as a coarser version of human beings.

MOUSE

When reading tea leaves, interpret a mouse as presaging financial loss or robbery. However, if you see one in real life, supposedly you will be happy in love.

OX
Tea leaves: hard work, often for no recognition.

The ox manifests yet another aspect of the cosmic forces at work, and in Ceremonial Magic, of agriculture and the earth. Since medieval times the ox represented Mother Earth, whose feminine "virtues" were submissiveness, patience, and self-sacrifice. In contrast to the lion and bull that represent the light, the ox signifies darkness, a logical association with the deep recesses of the earth.

PEACOCK
Tea leaves: riches; an estate; a wealthy marriage; vanity.

Peacocks, which still grace the lawns of some European manors and castles, capture images of immortality and the incorruptible soul. In Hindu myth, the eye-like patterns on the peacock's blue wings represent the stars in the sky; hence, our highest aspirations. In Ireland, screaming peacocks are thought to forecast rain. Christian symbology claims that moulting peacocks which reclothe again in splendor, imitate the resurrection of the body.

PHOENIX

Long before it became the name for a city in Arizona, the mythological phoenix was a compelling talisman in Oriental cultures. The Chinese believed that this bird lived for over five hundred years, built its own funeral pyre of dried grass in the desert, and proceeded to flap its wings over the fire until it was consumed by the flames. Then it arose, resurrected from the ashes. "Feng Huang," as they called the peacock, was regarded as a talisman for rebirth, longevity, and domestic tranquility. The phoenix became the emblem for empire, showing peace, prosperity, and benevolence.

On the other hand, the Japanese associate the bird with obedience, fidelity, justice, and rectitude.

SERPENT
Tea leaves: someone is plotting against the inquirer; vicious hatred.

The East Indians perceive the snake as a symbol of eternity, because it renews itself by casting off its old skin and assuming a new one. The ancient Greeks extrapolated from this concept the idea of healing, and entwined two serpents into what was to become the emblem of medical science.

In Egypt, the serpent was sculpted on the headdresses of royalty to show that the king was blessed with divine power, wisdom, and energy. However, it also became a sign of evil when Set assumed the form of a snake in order to escape the terrible vengeance of Horus. And of course in the Bible, the serpent is equated with temptation, destruction, and fall from grace, because it persuaded Eve to eat the apple in the Garden of Eden.

For talismanic purposes, the serpent brings the boons of longevity, good health, wisdom, and vitality to the wearer. It is especially lucky for teachers and doctors. To have a snake as a house pet is said to bring good fortune, and more practically, rid the house of rats!

SPIDER
Tea leaves: self-determination; cunning; good luck; when combined with dots, monetary gain.

The spider's web, which spirals to a central point where the arachnid makes its lair, is a personification of the universe. Some see in the spider a sign of transmutation because it weaves its web in the same way that it is perceived that human destiny is entwined. Others believe it to be a symbol of industrious labor.

Still others consider spiders to be creepy-crawly things, and have developed superstitions about them to mask their fears. One of these tales goes like this: if you see a spider in the morning, it is said you will come to grief; if at noon, you will find reason to be anxious; if at night, you will lose money.

VULTURE

Tea leaves: robbery; danger; someone in authority feels enmity toward the inquirer.

This bird was not always maligned as today. Because the vulture feeds on carrion, nowadays the bird is seen as a sign of death. However, in ancient Egypt, *Ner-t*, was revered as a symbol of Isis' motherly love and the ability to preserve humans from harm. The mother goddess assumed the form of a vulture when she went in search of her son, Horus. In hieroglyphics, the vulture spread its protective wings over temples and tombs. As a talisman, the bird delivered the wearer from scorpion bites, and brought both the living and the dead safety from evil as well as the stamina and fierceness of Isis.

EGYPTIAN TALISMANS

Egyptians were quite fond of talismans. Their charms were so elegantly conceived and designed, and the symbolic values of such universal appeal that today they continue to inspire us. Nowadays, they even are worn by those who have little or no knowledge of the concepts they express. Among the almost endless list of Egyptian charms are the following samples:

ANKH

A combination of a cross and the hieroglyph, *ru*, meaning "mouth," "gateway," and "creative power." The ankh demonstrates the dominion of spirit over matter, and grants life, love, power, and knowledge.

BUCKLE OF ISIS

Known as *tjet*, it represents the blood of Isis, and confers her strength, goodwill, and protection. The buckle is said to unlock hidden recesses and reveal secrets.

COLLAR

The collar was thought to free the deceased from the fetters binding their bodies and souls to the material plane.

NEFER

Often wrought in carnelian, it depicts a lute, and endows the wearer with youth, beauty, fortitude, graciousness, and good luck.

SCARAB

The lowly scarab, or beetle, patiently collects dung, lays an egg in it, and rolls it into a ball. Under the influence of the sun and moisture, the egg matures, and a new life is born. In these motions performed by this bug, the Egptians drew a parallel with the movement of the sun across the sky, which brought light and life to the world. Thus, the scarab represents transformation and creation, and as a talisman, embodies the virtue of fortitude and eternal life.

SHEN

This circle resting on a horizontal line symbolizes eternity and the bounty and power of the sun-god.

Egyptians also struck talismans in the shapes of animals. Some, like the frog, vulture, and cow, you have already met. Others include the hippopotamus, ram, bull, cat, jackal, crocodile, and pig.

Geometrical Forms

Geometrical designs and other simple shapes were a way for ancient people to cogently express complex symbols. With a few marks from a stylus or other writing implements, they communicated the meanings to others. In this way the runestones developed from a set of symbolic concepts into a script.

CRESCENT

Tea leaves: financial security; yearning for freedom; travel to a faraway land; an exotic stranger.

Symbol of the moon goddess, the crescent bestows on the wearer her blessings, and guards against misfortune.

CROSS

Tea leaves: protection.

Renowned as the emblem of Christianity, the cross in one form or another, predates Christianity by thousands of years.

Different types of crosses are: the tau cross, or *crux commissa*, found most frequently in the catacombs of Rome; maltese, or coptic, rayed cross; Greek, or equilateral cross; solar cross, representing the four quarters of heaven; St. Andrews cross, or *crux dessicata*; Latin cross, or *crux inmissa*, cross of Christ; Lorainne cross, the emblem of the Knights Hospitallers.

Among other ideas, the cross symbolizes protection, the four cardinal points, and dominion of spirit over matter. In runic divination, a cross in the form of an "x" means sacrifice. It was considered of such high amuletory value in ancient Greece that molds were made in the form of a cross and stamped into bread. Some cultures still serve hot crossed buns around Eastertime.

HEXAGRAM

The hexagram, or shield of Solomon, adds one more point to the pentagram's star. Viewed from another perspective, the shield is composed of two triangles, one pointing upward, and the other downward. The upward-pointing triangle represents good, truth, wisdom, fire, creation, spirit, the holy trinity, etc., while the downward-pointing triangle depicts evil, falsehood, folly, water, destruction, the material world, the devil, etc.

The Jews consider Solomon a great prophet, protector, and sage, and link the hexagram to him because the upward-pointing triangle is judged to denote the triumph of spirit over matter, a concept which according to the Hebrews, this king embodied.

It is also a symbol of the manifestation of the will on the material plane. For these reasons, the hexagram is a potent protective amulet and a talisman that grants the wearer immense powers. Qabalists developed a series of talismanic hexagrams (and pentagrams as well), which are explained in works like MacGregor Mathers' *The Greater Key of Solomon*, and *The Grimoire of Armadel*.

STAR

Tea leaves: good fortune.

The star is a symbol of the Moon goddess, and as a talisman, bestows on the wearer the blessings of the goddess, and guards against misfortune.

SWASTIKA

The swastika, or "fire wheel," is an ancient symbol, dating back to Neolithic times. It is a universal symbol, appearing in cultures as diverse as the American Indians and Tibetans, and even is found on ancient Scottish stone monuments. Although the Nazis perverted its meaning to their own nefarious purposes, the swastika's positive significance, which has evolved over thousands of years, is too potent to eradicate.

The true meaning of this emblem involves the representation of the four quarters of the universe set into motion, and the male and female principles. Talismanically, these virtues are translated into good luck and health, dominion, and increased wealth.

Miscellaneous Symbols

Other popular talismans not included in the above categories follow:

BELL

Tea leaves: a wedding.

Hebrew women sewed them into the hems of their skirts to drive away evil spirits. Gypsies still tie them to their horses for the same reason. During the hippie movement of the 1960's, flower children wore bells as a sign of peace and love.

CORNUCOPIA

Also known as the horn of plenty, it is a symbol of fruitfulness and prosperity. In mythology, it is said that the daughter of the king of Crete always kept Zeus supplied with good and abundant milk that she obtained from his goats. As a reward, the god bestowed on her the goat's horn so that she would never lack anything.

KEY

Tea leaves: a mystery.

A talisman designed in this shape is said to confer knowledge and prudence on the wearer, and open the door to the unknown. The key is associated with Janus, god of the threshold, to whom was attributed the invention of locks, doors, and gates, and to Jana, who presided over childbirth.

KNOT

Tea leaves: achievement.

Tied into childrens' clothes to avert the evil eye, knots defend against disruption, bind lovers, and solidify sacred bonds. Avoid wearing one during childbirth and death so that the spirit may be free to enter or leave the body as it pleases.

Inscriptive Talismans

An inscriptive talisman consists of a design called a sigil that represents a planetary force, or lettering of symbolic value that is painted, written, carved, burned, welded, or otherwise fixed on an object. The substance either can possess an inherent talismanic value, or be instilled with these properties by a Witch or Magician.

When the inscription is written on a piece of fine-quality paper or parchment (synthetic or genuine sheepskin), it is called a seal. Write seals with dove's blood ink for Positive Magic, dragon's blood ink for Negative or Protective Magic, or with the appropriately colored ink, pencil, or crayon to attract the desired planetary force.

If you wish to inscribe a talisman with a secret motto, use invisible ink following this recipe. Combine 95% distilled water and 5% cobalt and chloride. The ink is revealed by heating the paper.

Types of seals include the seal of Solomon, holy pentacles consecrated to numerous angelic forces and planets, Pennsylvania Dutch hex signs, sigils derived from the Sixth and Seventh Books of Moses, The Greater and Lesser Keys of Solomon, and other ancient holy books of occult knowledge, symbols of the four elements and spirit, planetary power symbols and number squares (for a detailed explanation of what these symbols and squares consist, why, and how they work, read Israel Regardie, *How to Make and Use Talismans*), Gnostic sigils, shields belonging to Christian saints, Voodoo veves, and Macumba and Candomble' *pontos riscados* (signs of the spirits and gods, scratched into dirt or sand. For a discussion of some of these symbols and illustrations, see *Pomba-Gira*, by Teixeira A. Neto and translated by Carol L. Dow, Technicians of the Sacred, 1992).

Often inscriptive talismans are written in magical or universal alphabets like Enochian, Hebrew, Egyptian hieroglyphics, and angelic alphabets.

Some popular inscriptive talismans and their meanings follow:

ABRACADABRA
Grants immunity against disease and other misfortune.

AGLA
The first letters of the words, "Ateh Gebur le-Olahm Adonai," meaning "thou art mighty forever, o Lord."

TETRAGRAMMATON
Derived from JHVH (Jehovah) meaning, "he that is and shall be." It delivers the wearer from enemies and bestows peace and harmony.

IAO
A Gnostic inscription meaning "the ineffable name of god."

AUM
Three Sanscrit letters signifying "creator, preserver, destroyer/transformer."

Herbal Sachets

A popular talisman is an herbal sachet, which is a powdered potpourri of dried flowers, herbs, leaves, and roots, plus perfume oils and a fixative. Place the sachet in a bag fashioned from a three-inch square of cotton or silk cloth, sew into the shape of a bag, and tie with ribbon, yarn, or thread. Alternatively, substitute a mojo bag, which is a small, red flannel bag, made to carry talismans. Wear the sachet around your neck or wrist, or carry it in your pocket or purse. You can make the sachet bag more elaborate by embroidering or painting it with appropriate symbols such as astrological or planetary signs, or any of the aforementioned figures in this chapter.

To give the sachet more body, add the powdered botanicals and oils to a sachet base. Do not use pure talcum powder as a base if you intend to add perfume oils, as talcum does not absorb these well. Cornstarch absorbs oils fairly well and is better to breathe than talcum powder.

To make a sachet base, place one part sandalwood, orris root powder, rosewood powder, or redwood powder in a bowl. Add powdered herbal ingredients in the amounts you require to achieve a particular scent, and oils. If you did not use orris root powder in the base, add one-half teaspoonful now as a fixative. Mix in nine parts cornstarch. Add natural dye or food coloring last, if desired. Use any combination of herbs described in chapter 7 chosen to achieve your purpose. Here are a few recipes to serve as models.

LOVE MAGNET SACHET

To 1/4 cup base, add 1 tablespoon rosebuds, 2 teaspoons musk crystals, 1/2 teaspoon peppermint, 1/2 teaspoon rose oil, 1/4 teaspoon light musk oil, 2 drops peppermint oil. The peppermint activates the spell.

LUCK O' THE IRISH SACHET

To 1/4 cup base, add 1 teaspoon comfrey, 2 teaspoons sage, 1/4 teaspoon hyssop, 1/2 teaspoon mint, 2 teaspoons clover oil.

MIND-READER SACHET

To 1/4 cup base, add 1 tablespoon lemon and orange peel, 1 teaspoon lavender flowers, 1/2 teaspoon hyssop, 1 teaspoon lemon verbena, 1/2 teaspoon sandalwood oil, 1/4 teaspoon narcissus oil.

WINGS OF HEALING SACHET

To 1/4 cup base, add 1 teaspoon rosemary leaves, 1 teaspoon thyme, 1 teaspoon sage, 1/2 teaspoon violet oil, 1/4 teaspoon bergamot oil.

Chapter 6:

Talismanic Ritual To Integrate The Intellect Into The Whole Self

Full Moon in Aquarius
Perform at noon or midnight

This chapter shows how to incorporate the information you have learned about talismans into a ritual. It includes an herbal talisman and the consecration of a stone, as well as some herbs to enclose inside the talismanic bag. The ritual requires anointing and charging a gemstone and accompanying herbs as a talisman. I chose aquamarine because it is the gem of the mystic, seer, and ocean wanderer. This stone is ruled by Uranus and Aquarius, and confers upon the wearer intuition, wisdom, and clairvoyance. Moreover, it synthesizes these powers into a harmonious whole.

In this ritual you invoke Odin because he represents the synthesis of two aspects of the god that are crucial to this rite. The first is Kronos, the original sky deity, symbol of fertility of body and mind, and protector and sewer of the seed. Yet Kronos was overthrown by Zeus, the new lord of the skies, who through his ability to control the elements, particularly lightning and thunder, heralded the golden age.

Odin integrates both these concepts into one form. It is the great god, Odin, who sacrifices himself on the World Tree, Yggdrasill, in order to obtain the runes of knowledge for humanity. Because of his sacrifice, Odin is privileged with understanding the secrets of the cosmos.

Items Required

To perform this ritual you will need: two sky blue altar candles anointed with Aquarius oil, astral candles of the participants anointed with their zodiac oils, candle holders; Aquarius incense, coal, burner, matches; Druidic Holy Oil to anoint the third eye of the participants and the talisman; Aquarius-blue altar cloth; Vayu tattva (bright blue circle) and the tarot card, the Hierophant, reversed, for meditation; consecrated salt and water; aquavit liqueur and crystal goblet for the libation to Odin; aquamarine stone, pinches of frankincense, myrrh, southernwood, spikenard, and a mojo bag.

Organize the ritual space, consecrate the salt and water, light the candles, and anoint the third eye of the participants.

Meditation

Prior to the ritual, and to place yourself into a proper frame of mind, the participants may meditate on improving the intellect, finding innovative approaches to challenges, developing the imagination, or synthesis.

Aquarius is ruled by Uranus, the elusive, remote planet that symbolizes motion, changeability, and electrical energy. As you meditate on your purpose in this rite, I ask you to focus on the Vayu tattva and the image of the tarot card, the Hierophant reversed. These symbols remind us to dig deep within our beings to root out anything from our lives that resembles complacency, smugness, or stasis. Complacency is a warning of submission of the life force to the material, and smugness brings death to the soul. If we do not constantly move and change, we cannot evolve to fulfill our true destinies.

At the same time, we realize that undirected motion also exhausts our energies and evaporates into stasis. So in your meditation, I ask that you pursue a way to synthesize the motivating force of your intellect into your entire being — mind, psyche, soul and spirit — in order to achieve your highest aims.

The following adaptation of a poem by Charles Lamb dedicated to the element, Air, may help you set the tone of your reverie:

"I could laugh to hear the midnight wind,
That, rushing on its way with careless sweep
Scatters the ocean waves. And I could weep
Like to a child. For now to my raised mind
On wings of wind comes wild-eyed Phantasy,
And her rude visions give severe delight."

Opening of the Circle

After a while, the Priestess rings the bell to arouse the participants from their reverie, lights the incense, astral candles of the participants, and the candle in the south, and opens the Circle using the Lesser Banishing and Invoking Pentagram rituals (described in *Web of Light*.) It is important to the success of this rite that the participants link in by visualizing the ray of electric-blue light that the Priestess draws down through her Athame to protect and illuminate the Circle. This dazzling light represents the essence of the planetary forces to be invoked.

Also, as a reminder, the Athame, or ritual dagger with which the Priestess draws the Circle, is the primary symbol of the element, Air, and the representation of her life force.

Invocation to Odin

The Priestess faces the altar and invokes:

"Great god Odin,
Claimer of the holy runes,
We invoke you to fly to this Circle of Light.
Enfold us in your cobalt cloak,
Transport us to the mantle of the noonday (midnight) sky
To the loftiest realms of the universe.
Let us behold through your blazing blue eye
The secret depths that only you can choose to show us.
Riding the trapeze in breathless flight,

Shot from earth
Angel earth
Venturing adventure we travel.
Force creating form
Form forming force
Stability in motion
Spiral to heaven
Neither heaven or earth,
Between the worlds suspended.
O thou shaper of worlds,
Destiny in movement
Catapult us into
Change without strings
Risking it all we fly
Netless
To Odin."

Consecration of the Talisman

The participants bring forth their aquamarines and the herbs.
Each participant places a small amount of the dried herbs in a mojo
bag while the Priestess circumscribes on the ground with blue glitter
or with her Athame the symbol of a pentagram within a circle. Before
the participants place their stones in the center of the Circle, each
holds the stone in her/his left hand, cups the right hand over it, and
announces either aloud or privately the talismanic purpose of the
gem. Then she/he blows on it three times, and places it in the center
of the pentagram. The Priestess purifies and consecrates the stones
by passing them through the symbols of the four elements (incense
smoke, red Quarter candle, water, and salt), and then anoints them
with Druidic Holy oil.

The participants sit in a circle around the gems, holding hands,
and recite the following chant:

"LIGHT SHINE FORTH"

As they chant, they visualize that they are creating a ring of
electric-blue light that encircles them, and gradually rise above them

forming a cone of power. When the chant culminates, they let go of hands and direct the cone of energy into their heads, down their shoulders and out their fingertips to the stones. The aquamarines should sparkle with the charging energy. If this rite is performed correctly, the stones may feel warm to the touch as each participant picks her/his own and encloses it in the herb-filled mojo bag.

Ritual Libation

The Priestess pours aquavit into a crystal goblet, and purifies and consecrates the libation. She extends her Athame over the cup and says:

"Fragrance of the fruits of this earth, by the power of this sacred blade, I exorcise you of all impurities. May you be fresh and unsullied as the purity of our intentions."

She immerses the tip of the dagger into the liquid and recites:

"Draught of inspiration, you who sparks our creative juices and helps us perceive not one way only, but all ways, be consecrated. Bring happiness to those who partake of your rich and vital essence. May you ever dignify the god, whose life blood you incarnate."

The Priestess spills some of the liqueur on the ground, to the left, right, and center of the altar, and calls,

"For you, Odin, the first taste of the drink that honors you."

Then she passes the goblet around the Circle for all to imbibe. The participants may verbally share any insights experienced during the meditation and rite, or simply sit back and enjoy the feeling of unity with the god.

Closing the Circle

The Priestess closes the Circle using the Lesser Banishing Pentagram Ritual, and thanks Uriel, Archangel of Uranus and Aquarius, the sylphs, elemental spirits of Air, and any unseen guests that have been attracted to the energy focus of the rite, and particularly Odin, for attending the Circle.

The ritual is ended. Empty the salt and water on the ground and thoroughly clean and put away all ritual equipment immediately. It is unwise to let the electrical charge of Uranus energy linger in the area.

Chapter 7:
A Witch's Herbal

In the past, Witches believed that Hecate, the goddess of Witchcraft, revealed to them the secrets of herbs. Witches believed that the Wise Crone had blessed them with this knowledge so that they could cure humankind of all ills, and eventually bring about a new and perfect world, whom many called Avallon. This privilege was also deemed a great responsibility.

Today Witches still strive toward this goal. Whether or not they still believe in the tale of Hecate's gift, they approach the study of herbs, known to them as wortcunning, with reverence. Each time a Witch handles an herb, she thinks of its symbolic value, and in a sense, transforms the botanical into a sacred object and living force.

Witches reserve one day during the year when they honor the healing power of herbs. This occurs on the Summer Solstice, when the herbal essences coursing through plants are at their most concentrated levels.

As the coven gathers around the Solstice needfire, each member brings forth a personally significant herb, explains its meaning, and drops it into the fire. The fragrant smoke wafts the private petitions to the gods (or, if you prefer, dispels the energy through the cosmos), so that her/his force of will is able to bring about the changes she/he requests. It is a stirring rite, and a fine method of putting yourself in contact with the natural world. It is also a good way to become familiar with herbal attributes and uses.

As you peruse the following herbal, you will notice that it is organized to give both medicinal and magical information about each botanical. The plant name is followed by alternative names by which it is known, as these differ from region to region, and English-speaking country to country.

The names are followed by associations, which usually are planetary and astrological. Back in the heyday of the Doctrine of Signatures, each plant was assigned an association according to its characteristics and action. This information helps you understand the magical properties of each botanical.

Also, because Witches perform many planetary rites and prescribe herbal medicine according to the astrological sign of the patient, or the sign governing the symptoms of the ailment, it is valuable to have these associations at hand as a reference. If you need to study or review the planets, I suggest you read the relevant chapters in *Secrets of a Witch's Coven, Web of Light,* or Israel Regardie's *The Art of True Healing.*

Next comes a short description of each plant to help put you on the right road toward identifying it. Given space limitations in the book and the fact that the herbal concentrates on magical uses of herbs, the descriptions are general. I suggest you carry along a plant identification book when harvesting plants in the wild. Books filled with pictures of plants are most suitable. Many benign plants resemble poisonous botanicals. When in doubt, do not pick a questionable herb. Also, never remove more than one-third of a stand of botanicals in the wild to give them a chance to bounce back.

Following the description, a paragraph or two explains medicinal action claimed by herbalists. Appendix I: Medical Terms will help you understand the technical words used throughout the herbal.

Each segment closes with alleged occult meanings of the botanicals and how to use them in rituals. Herbs that predominate in perfumery and incense-making are described further in *Witch's Brew.* Happy wortcunning!

ABSINTHE
Names: *Artemisia absinthium,* **Wormwood, Old Woman, Madderwort, Green Ginger.**
Associations: Isis, Mercury, Artemis, Venus, Mars, Scorpio.

Absinthe is a bitter herb, known world-wide in temperate climates as a moth and flea repellant, and as the signature ingredient of absinthe liqueur. The plant's gray stem is covered with fine hairs. The leaves are grayish green, and the flowers are small and yellow.

This botanical is prized as an antipyretic, antiseptic, stomachic, anthelmintic, emmenagogue, and possible narcotic.

Sprinkle the dried leaves under your bed to draw a lover. Burn the leaves together with sandalwood to communicate with spirits of the dead. Scatter them among your linens and clothing to rid yourself of evil influences. The tea allegedly is an aphrodisiac.

AGRIMONY
Names: *Agrimonia eupatoria*, Bur Marigold, Cocklebur (so named for the bristly fruit), Church Steeples (named after the shape of the little yellow flowers), stickwort.
Associations: Jupiter, Cancer, Sagittarius.

This perennial grows two- to- three- feet high along the roadside. The brownish-yellow flowerheads smell a bit like cedar when burned.

In herbal medicine, the plant is valued as an alterative, antibiotic, febrifuge, hepatic tonic, vulnerary, antipyretic, cathartic, diuretic, astringent and anti-inflammatory. It cures blemishes when applied externally. Prepare agrimony tea to moderate the chills and fever associated with flu. Apply it in a poultice to stings, wounds, and sore muscles.

Carry this botanical in a magical pouch to defeat villains. Cast sleep spells with agrimony by placing it under the pillow of the recipient, who will fall into a deep, dreamless stupor.

ALFALFA
Names: *Medicago sativa* (meaning "sowed by the Medicans," the ancient Persians who first cultivated the crop), Buffalo Herb, Chilean Clover, Lucerne, Purple Medic. The name of this plant from the pea family comes into English from Spanish via Arabic. Both cultures believed that by feeding their horses alfalfa fodder, their steeds would achieve fantastic speed, strength, and endurance. In Arabic the common name means "Father of All Foods."
Associations: Gemini, Libra, Jupiter.

The sprouts of this hardy, grassy perennial are used as a fodder. Alfalfa also is a ready source of potassium, magnesium, phosphorus, calcium, vitamins A, B, C, and K, organic salts, and essential enzymes. For centuries it has been used as a soil- improving crop.

Alfalfa's attributes include its use as a nutritive tonic, antipyretic, alterative, and hemostatic. Drink an infusion of the leaves with other herbs like fennel and guaraná to lose weight. Alfalfa is used to lower the blood pressure. The herb in the bath hastens recovery from an illness.

This herb is alleged to confer good luck, longevity, and a youthful appearance. Keep it in your cupboard to insure your household against poverty.

ALOE
Names: *Aloe vera,* **Aloes.**
Associations: Saturn, Venus, Mars, Sagittarius.

A succulent perennial of the lily family, aloe is grown in Curaçao and Barbados, where it blooms most of the year. The narrow leaves are prickly edged and fleshy with juice, which when added to shampoo, helps prevent hair loss. The juice is also a valued skin repairer in face and body lotions. *Lignum aloes,* often confused with aloe because of the similarity of the Latin name, refers to a fragrant wood used to scent incense.

A staple of the herbalist's medicine chest, aloe works as an emmenagogue, emollient, demulcent, laxative, vulnerary, vermifuge, and carminative. Add it to lotions to relieve poison ivy sting and rough, detergent hands. Apply it directly to cuts and bruises. The juice helps cure eczema, female problems, kidney and liver, and gall bladder disorders, diarrhea, tonsillitis, headache, and burns from radiation. Avoid using it during pregnancy.

In the realm of Magic, aloe procures love, helps make a person attractive to the opposite sex, and invokes demons. The Egyptians considered it an emblem of their religious faith, and hung it over their doorways as a sign that the dweller had made a religious pilgrimage. In the language of flowers, the plant symbolizes "grief."

ANGELICA
Names: *Angelica archangelica,* **Root of the Holy Ghost.**
Associations: Sun, Venus, Michael, Leo.

A fragrant, leafy plant of the carrot family that flourishes in cool climates, the thick stem can grow as tall as a small tree. Unfortunately, I have only succeeded in cultivating them as high as my waist in the dry climate where I live. Use the roots, leaves, and seeds. The latter are the signature ingredient of the liqueur, Chartreuse. Candy the thick, hollow stems for a sweet treat.

Angelica is a diuretic, stomachic, stimulant, tonic, emmenagogue, carminative, diaphoretic, expectorant, alterative for the circulation and for when the body needs an extra push, stomachic, and diuretic. An infusion of the seeds relieves flatulence. The tea made from the root is an aromatic stimulant and tonic that combats nausea, and helps cure coughs, colds, pleurisy, colic, and urinary tract infections.

Legend has it that angelica was revealed to humanity by the Archangel Michael in a dream as a remedy against contagious diseases, poison, and plague. Lost to us now is the reason behind the chanting ritual that in Eastern Europe used to accompany the herb into town for sale on market day. It is a powerful uncrossing herb because angelica is said to neutralize evil. Chew the root or sprinkle it in the corners of your house to avoid Black Magic and ill health. In the language of flowers the plant symbolizes "inspiration."

ANISE
Names: *Pimpinella anisum,* **Sweet Cumin, Aniseed.**
Associations: Mercury, Jupiter, Moon.

An umbelliferous annual of the carrot family, the fruit are used to flavor soups, cheesescakes, and liqueurs. Anise and fennel look and taste very much alike. Spread the oil on fish lures and traps for small animals (especially mice). Be aware that the oil is lethal to pigeons. Star anise (*Illicum verum*), which smells and tastes like anise, is a small tree indigenous to China.

As a carminative, stimulant, diuretic, antiseptic, and expectorant, anise helps ease digestion of pork and beef and checks flatulence. The herb contains properties that break up mucus in pectoral infections and ease hard, dry coughs. Chew the licorice-tasting fruit as a breath freshener.

Anise is a favorite magical sachet ingredient. Inhale the fruit crushed in Meditation incense in order to purify yourself in mind and body in preparation to work Magic, curb alcohol and nicotine addictions, and facilitate psychic development and clairvoyance. Anise is alleged to avert the evil eye and encourage visions.

ARNICA
Names: *Arnica montana,* Leopard's-bane, Mountain Tobacco.
Associations: Jupiter, Saturn.

This hairy-leafed perennial that grows in high country meadow and valleys, has golden-colored aromatic flowers reminiscent of marigolds. In fact, the flowers sometimes are found for sale adulterated with marigolds.

It is a poisonous plant that irritates the stomach and dramatically increases blood pressure. For these reasons I strongly discourage its internal use. Nonetheless, in the past some herbalists recommended it to relieve epilepsy, nerve shock, and sea sickness. Apply externally with care a tincture of the flowers to sprains, bruises, and wounds.

Carrying this botanical is reputed to protect travellers from the attacks of wild beasts.

ASAFOETIDA
Names: *Ferula foetida,* Devil's Dung, Food of the Gods.
Associations: Moon, Saturn.

An umbelliferous herb with pale green and yellow flowers and a bristly, fleshy root, the plant reaches up to seven-feet high. The milky fruit has a fetid odor and a bitter, acrid taste. Nonetheless, it is used by East Indians and Asians as a condiment.

Asafoetida is known principally as a carminative to counteract flatulence, colic, asthma, and bronchitis. Eat it with gypsum to gain weight.

Persians believed asafoetida stimulated the brain. Wear it around your neck in a sachet to ward off disease and other negative vibrations. Combined in a paste with garlic and rubbed on your lover's feet, it is said to keep her/him true.

BALM OF GILEAD
Names: *Abies balsamea,* Balsam of Gilead, Silver Pine, Silver Fir.
Associations: Sun, Venus Jupiter.

The sticky, resin-covered buds are the product of a fragrant tree of the pine family, long known by the North American Indians for its medicinal value. The buds and needles are a festive addition to Winter Solstice incense.

Balsam fir is an antiseptic, aromatic, stimulant, tonic, and diuretic. It assuages pains in the stomach, lungs, and kidneys, counteracts the effects of colds and coughs, and alleviates gout and rheumatism.

The buds of the poplar tree *(Populus niger)* are frequently substituted in incense-making and spellwork, as they both have the same magical properties.

Wear the buds of either tree in a sachet as an amulet for protection against hexes and to mend your broken heart. In the Bible it is written that the Queen of Sheba brought Gilead buds to Judea as a present to King Solomon.

Steep the buds in wine, dry them, and string them into a necklace to draw love. It is thought that if you coat your fingers with the sticky resin, you can pass through fire without being burned. The buds also are an ingredient of solar incenses such as Helios and Egyptian incenses like Jewel of the Nile.

BASIL

Names: *Ocimum basilicum;* variations include Culinary Sweet Basil, and Purple Ornamental Basil. The name is derived from the basilisk, a mythological dragon-like creature.
Associations: Mars, Scorpio, Jupiter, Krishna, Vishnu, Saturn.

A popular herb found in many kitchen gardens, it is a bushy annual with inch-long, toothed, oval to elliptical leaves and small, white or purple flowers that look somewhat like mint. The aroma of the crushed leaves is pungently spicy and peppery.

The flowers are a carminative, antipyretic, stimulant, alterative, diuretic, emmenagogue, and nervine. Chewing the leaves relieves intestinal gas. The aroma dispels melancholy.

Hang a sprig of dried basil above the main door of your house to prevent evil from entering. Wear it in your hair to attract a lover. In Egypt, bouquets of basil were placed in the hands of the dead instead of lilies. In times gone by, basil was highly regarded as a protective herb that was charged to invoke wild beasts.

Spread basil on the doorway and threshold of a store to attract customers and deter thieves and vandals. Chew the leaves to increase your fertility.

Basil is a reputed aphrodisiac and in medieval England was thought to cure venereal disease; hence its old name, "wylde times." The Portuguese thought basil symbolized boldness and could enable a person to fly.

BETONY

Names: *Stachys betonica*, Wood Betony, Woundwort, Bishopswort. The plant is believed to be named for Beronie, a woman who was said to have been healed by Christ. In Celtic herbology, the name means "good for the head," and in ancient Britain the plant was reputed to cure headaches.
Associations: Mars, Sagittarius, Jupiter, Aries.

This woodland plant was "discovered" in mythology by Chiron the Centaur as a substitute for black tea. It is a slender, square-stemmed two-foot high plant with two-lipped purplish-red flowers. Betony yields a yellow dye and makes a fine incense base.

At one time, betony was believed to be a panacea, and the Saxon Herbals claimed that it healed body and soul. People thought that injured animals sought it out to cure their wounds, and that if two snakes were placed inside a ring of betony, they would kill each other.

It is an alterative, analgesic, nervine, parasiticide, and a tonic and nervine when taken in combination with other herbs. Betony also is used as a tobacco substitute combined with eyebright and coltsfoot leaves. Mix it with marjoram and eyebright as a snuff to cure headaches.

Betony can be fashioned into a Druidic amulet to protect against terrifying visions and evil spirits. It also supposedly fortifies the body and spirit. Wear it around your neck to keep safe from harm when visiting churchyards.

BISTORT

Names: *Polygonum bistorta*, Adderwort, Dragonwort, Easter Ledger, Snakeweed.
Associations: Cancer, Saturn.

The characteristically twisted roots of this slender stemmed plant provide inspiration for some of its popular names, and is probably why in days gone by in accordance with the Doctrine of Signatures the herb was considered a cure for snake bite. A hardy member of the buckwheat family, bistort is covered with clusters of pink or white flowers from May through August. The leaves can be eaten like spinach.

It is a strong vegetable astringent that effectively checks internal and external bleeding. Since the plant contains starch and grows profusely in northern climes, it has been consumed during hard times in Iceland and Russia.

Bistort is effective against diarrhea, cholera, dysentery, and stomach, nose and lung bleeding. It alleviates hemorrhoids, hypermenorrhea, ulcerated gums, and insect stings. Formerly (and with no scientific basis) the plant was thought to help women conceive and retain a fetus. Around the Lake District of Western England some women may still eat a bistort pudding at Eastertime to aid conception.

Add it to incense to promote psychic visions. Bistort allegedly grants the user power on the astral plane. Steep and strain 1 tablespoonful of bistort in a pint of barley water, and add it to your floor wash to chase away poltergeists.

BLADDERWRACK

Names: *Fucus vesiculosus*, Bladder Fucus, Kelpware, Rockweed, Seawrack.
Associations: Jupiter, Lir, the Mermaids, Morgana, all the ocean deities.

This seaweed looks like little bladders that stick like suction cups to rocks.

As a good source of iodine, bladderwrack is a remedy for goiter. Traditionally it was used to cure obesity stemming from hypothyroid. Use it as a liniment to ease rheumatism. It also soothes throat irritations.

Throw bladderwrack into the ocean when petitioning the sea deities. Use it in rituals to find treasure buried at sea, or to insure a safe journey by water.

BLESSED THISTLE

Names: *Cnicus benedictus*, Holy Thistle, Spotted Thistle (so- called because during the Middle Ages the plant was thought to cure smallpox and other "spotty" diseases).
Associations: Mars, Aries.

This annual thistle grows on a hairy brown stem. Its spry, yellow flowers bloom from May to August.

Traditionally this botanical is used as a tonic, galactogogue, stimulant, emmenagogue, emetic, alterative, and diaphoretic. It eases painful menstruation, shooting pains, fevers, pernicious anemia, jaundice, gallstones, and worms. The plant is touted by many herbalists as a natural contraceptive.

Blessed thistle is a traditional amulet against melancholy and plague. Add it to your bath water to win spiritual and financial blessings.

BLOODROOT

Names: *Sanguinaria canadensis,* Indian Paint, Red Puccoon, Redroot, Tetterwort.

Associations: Mars, the warrior gods of the North American Indians, Venus, Scorpio.

A poisonous plant of the poppy family found in woods, fields, and on river banks, it has a nauseating taste. The fleshy root is used by some American Indians as a dye. It is identified by its single white flower and pale green lobed leaf which sprouts from the reddish-orange rhizome.

The roots are a cathartic, expectorant, emmenagogue, and emetic. Traditionally the plant was used to cure bronchitis, dyspepsia, asthma, ringworm, eczema, skin cancer, and fungal growths. I do not recommend you prescribe this plant medicinally because it is strongly emetic and lowers the pulse rate dangerously. The root is so caustic it corrodes tissue.

Bloodroot's main magical virtue is as an amulet against evil spirits. Throw it on an enemy's doorstep to turn back wicked spells. Burn the powdered root for seven nights at midnight to purify your dwelling.

BONESET

Names: *Eupatorium perfoliatum,* Teasel, Ague Weed, Feverwort, Indian Sage, Thoroughwort, Crosswort. Contrary to its name, boneset does not help set bones. It received its name from the effective way it dealt with breakbone fever, which was common in the nineteenth century.

Associations: the *loas* of American Voodoo, Capricorn, Saturn.

Boneset grows in meadows, prairies and swamps in the southern United States. The plant displays flat-topped clusters of white flowerheads and wrinkled, hairy leaves and stems.

It is a stimulant, febrifuge, antispasmodic, nervine, antipyretic, diaphoretic, and laxative. The Pilgrims used this bitter herb to cure colds and fevers because it increases perspiration. It also stimulates the digestion when consumed as a bitter tea. Boneset infusions help reduce typhoid and yellow fevers. The herb can be employed as a skin ointment when mixed with vaseline.

It is a favorite herb for stuffing Voodoo dolls in order to throw back a curse. Anna Riva in her herbal recommends boneset in the following spell to curse one's enemy. As you burn the dried leaves, recite,

> "I alone will break your bone,
> You can no longer harm me,
> The harm you've done returns to you,
> As sure as sky turns blue." [11]

BORAGE

Names: *Borago officinalis*, Burridge, Bee Bread, Bugloss, Star-flower.

Associations: Jupiter, Cybele, Leo.

The purplish-blue, starlike flowers of this tall, fuzzy-leafed herb that flourishes in wastelands, (and multiplies rapidly in the garden) attract hoards of honeybees and make a tasty candied treat. The leaves provide an interesting salad green with a cool, cucumbery taste. The nitrate of potash content causes the flowers to spark and explode when burned, which when added to incense, increases the sense of drama in invocation rituals.

The herb is prized as an antipyretic, diuretic, emollient, and galactogogue. Drink a tea made from the leaves mixed with lemon, sugar and wine to cure a sore throat and restore your strength after a long illness. The tea also is good for lung disease. The herb's perspiration-producing properties help eliminate poisons from the body.

Borage makes an ideal herb for health rituals and talismans. The tea is said to lift the spirits and strengthen one's resolve.

BROOM

Names: *Cytisus scoparius*, **Broom Tops, Brownie, Genista, Irish Broom, Scotch Broom.**
Associations: Mars, Aries.

This stiffly branched shrub that grows in the desolate regions of Scotland, Ireland and France in former times was used as a household broom, hence the name. The plant has cheerful, yellow, pea-like flowers. It's medieval name, *Planta genista*, was taken up by a dynasty of English kings when Henry II adopted the plant as the heraldic symbol of his line, called the Plantagenet.

It is a poisonous botanical, no longer recommended for internal use, but which traditionally was used as a cathartic and diuretic.

Ward off negative Witchcraft by wearing broom flowers in your hair. Boil broom tops with salt, and sprinkle the water throughout the house to keep poltergeists at bay. Curiously, because it is so pretty, the shrub in full bloom is supposed to bring bad luck. As the saying goes, "If you sweep the house with a blossomed broom in May, you are sure to sweep the head of the house away."

On the other hand, if a stand of broom blossoms with many flowers it is said to harbinger prosperous times. In France, the plant is associated with humility. The flowers also have a reputation as tranquilizers and are a powerful magnet for love.

CALAMUS

Names: *Acorus calamus*, **Sedge, Sweet Flag, Flagroot, Sweetroot, Sweet Cane, Sweet Grass, Sweet Rush.**
Association: Sun.

This is a perennial herb that grows swordlike, lemony-smelling leaves resembling rushes. In times gone by, the leaves were strewn on the floors of farmhouses to sweeten the air. The cut root adds a sweet aroma to incense.

This poisonous botanical may cause tumors, so it is not recommended for internal use. However, traditionally, herbalists used the rhizome as an antispasmodic and stomachic. It is also added to lotions to relieve itchy skin.

The American Indians of the Northwest held pieces of the rhizome in their mouths during battle because they believed it increased their endurance and stamina. The herb is mentioned often in the Bible, but sometimes is confused with sweet grass. In Voodoo it is burned with Graveyard Dust as a controlling agent.

CAMPHOR
Name: *Cinnamomum camphora.*
Associations: Moon, Diana, Cancer.

Camphor is the white, crystalline gum of a 100-foot evergreen tree native to Japan and China that is prized as a moth repellant, especially when combined with wormwood. It is a key ingredient of lunar incense.

Internal use of this poisonous herb, fatal to infants, is discouraged. Herbalists of old attributed to it stimulant and nervine properties, and used it to prevent heart failure, colds, chills, and fatigue. Apply camphor gum externally to lessen the pain from rheumatism, neuralgia, inflammation of the heart, and poor circulation.

Camphor fulfills offertory and talismanic purposes when invoking the power of the Moon. In times of epidemic, some Voodoo practitioners wear a lump of camphor on a string around their necks to ward off disease.

CARAWAY
Name: *Carum carui.* **The name in Old English means "Care-away," and refers to the herb's soothing properties.**
Associations: Mercury, Saturn.

Caraway is a common culinary herb of the carrot family, similar to anise, dill, and fennel. The plant grows two-feet high and has white or yellow flowers and feathery, dusty green or turquoise leaves. The herb's long, tapered root often is confused with deadly water hemlock. The root is an aromatic in incenses. Since Roman times, caraway has been used to flavor cookies, bread, cake, soup, cabbage, cheese, and Kummel liqueur.

It is a carminative and mild stimulant to the digestion. Powder the seeds and make a poultice to reduce swelling from bruises. Chewing caraway seeds helps relieve intestinal gas.

Keep the seeds in your home to prevent your possessions from being stolen. It is alleged to keep lovers faithful, and to reveal if a lover is telling the truth. For this reason it makes a useful component of some love talismans. Sew the seeds into a small bag, and stuff it in your baby's pillow to keep your child free from harm. If you own poultry, feed them caraway seeds to keep them from straying from the barnyard.

CATNIP

Names: *Nepeta cataria*, **Catmint, Cat's-play.**
Associations: Venus, Mars, Mercury.

A strong-smelling botanical of the mint family, it grows easily in poor soil, and like most mints, spreads rapidly. The white to pinkish flowers form in tubular clusters atop square, branching stems.

The leaves of this three foot tall herb are a carminative, diaphoretic, antispasmodic, stimulant (especially for cats), tonic, nervine, and slight emmenagogue. It makes an excellent tea for nervous headaches. Catnip cures childrens' diarrhea, especially when used as an enema. Combined with lemon balm, marshmallow root, and licorice, it is good for baby's colic, irritability, and colds. Place the fresh leaves in a foot bath to relieve stuffiness and other cold symptoms. From personal experience, I can say that if you grow catnip, your feline friends will never desert you!

Because of its popularity with cats the plant is considered a key ingredient beneficial in rites to invoke Bast, the Egyptian cat goddess. A tea made from the leaves dispels nightmares. Strew catnip around the campsite to drive away snakes.

CAYENNE

Name: *Capsicum minimum.*
Association: Mars.

This red pepper is known best as a condiment for hot and spicy Mexican-style food; hence its name, which in Greek means "to bite."

Cayenne is beneficial as a stimulant, stomachic, rubefacient, antispasmodic, and hemostatic. It helps normalize blood circulation, and prevents diarrhea.

Use a pinch of this botanical to activate spells. Employ it in rites to increase sexual potency. Cayenne powder is a traditional ingredient in Hotfoot Powder, a Voodoo mixture said to cause someone to move away. Voodoo practitioners swear they can cause trouble between a man and a woman by combining cayenne powder, iron filings, flaxseed, gunpowder, and dirt taken from a graveyard, and throwing the mixture against the couple's house. To make the popular Flying Devil Oil, combine olive oil and cayenne pepper, and tint the mixture with red food coloring.

CHAMOMILE

Names: *Anthemis nobilis* **(Roman),** *Matricaria chamomilla* **(German chamomile), Camomile, Manzanilla. The name comes from a German word meaning "earth apple."**

Association: Sun. The Egyptians so believed in the powers of chamomile to cure influenza that they dedicated the plant to all their gods.

The apple-scented flowers of this bright, sturdy little herb resemble daisies. Several varieties exist, including German (good as a tea), Hungarian (the most bitter variety), Roman (the showy flowers are used in potpourri), and Egyptian (usually the cheapest). When planted near other plants, it helps them grow, and attracts beneficial insects to the garden. I make a hair rinse from the flowers and use it in the wintertime to add highlights to my blond hair.

Medicinal properties of this botanical include: antispasmodic, stomachic, tonic, anodyne, sedative, emmenagogue, nervine, carminative, and diaphoretic. A poultice of the flowers combined with poppy seeds reduces swellings and inflammations of muscles and gums. Chamomile flowers cure the pain from earache and neuralgia.

Chamomile is beneficial in spells to promote business and increase wealth, especially if you rinse your hands in the tea before beginning the business day or gambling. Use the flowers in spells to gain peace of mind. In medieval times, people strewed pathways with the cut herb or grew it along the roadside so that its apple-like aroma would release as passersby trod on it.

CHICORY

Names: *Cichorium intybus,* **Blue-sailors, Coffeeweed, Succory.**
Association: Uranus.

Since the sky-blue flowers open and close at the same time each day, chicory makes a perfect plant for a floral clock. According to the Doctrine of Signatures and Sympathetic Magic, this botanical strengthens failing eyesight.

Chicory makes a bitter, tangy seasoning for soups and stews. The long taproot thrives in terrain hostile to less hardy plants. The new leaves in a salad taste bitter like Belgian endive, which is a variety of chicory.

In herbal medicine it is used as a diuretic, laxative, and liver tonic. A poultice made from the crushed root reduces inflammations. Since roasted chicory root tastes somewhat like coffee but contains no caffeine, it makes an acceptable coffee substitute.

Legend has it that if you powder the root, add it to a Crossing incense, and burn it on nine consecutive nights while repeating your enemy's name, you will remove all the curses wrought by the offender. Another legend claims that if you cut it with a golden scythe at noon on July 25, the plant will make you invisible and help you open locked doors and chests...so mark your calendar! In the language of plants, this botanical stands for "frugality."

CINNAMON

Name: *Cinnamomum zeylanicum.*
Associations: Sun, Uranus.

This plant does not properly fall within the strict definition of an herb, as it is extracted from the inner bark of a medium-sized tropical tree. However, it is used widely in incense-making, perfumery and cookery. Cassia bark (*Cassia fistula*) has similar properties, but is not of as high a quality.

Cinnamon is an astringent, stimulant, antiseptic, carminative, and hemostatic. It stops hemorrhaging from the womb, and cures lower back pain, flatulence, vomiting, and diarrhea. Because the oil can burn the skin it should be used parsimoniously in fragrance crafting. It is possible to substitute allspice oil, but the results are not the same.

The spicy bark enjoys a reputation as an aphrodisiac in love potions. Bake a white apple cake with plenty of cinnamon and give a piece to the person you admire. She/he soon will be yours. Weave cinnamon sticks into wreaths as the Romans did to perfume and decorate their temples. Cinnamon is an occasional ingredient of money-draw incenses.

CINQUEFOIL

Names: *Potentilla reptans*, **Five Fingers Grass. The Latin name means "small and powerful."**
Associations: Jupiter, Mercury.

Cinquefoil is a pretty, creeping perennial of the rose family that spreads in runners like strawberries. The leaves also look like strawberry leaves, but unlike the strawberry, this plant bears a single five-petaled yellow flower.

It is an analgesic, astringent, antipyretic, and antihemorrhagic that stops nosebleeds. A decoction of the root cures mouth sores and fevers, and a tea made from the leaf stops diarrhea.

Five fingers grass is an important Voodoo herb used for miscellaneous purposes. By tradition, the leaf segments represent luck, money, wisdom, power, and love.

In medieval times the herb was a heraldic symbol on shields that indicated the knight had achieved self-mastery.

To drive away evil and destroy your enemies, baste a wax image of your enemy in wine that has been steeped with cinquefoil. If hung over the bed this botanical is reputed to banish negativity and nightmares. Add the leaves to your purification bath before performing rituals.

It is also an ingredient of love potions and good luck mojo bags.

CLOVE
Names: *Caryophyllus aromaticus, Syzygium aromaticum.*
Associations: Sun, Uranus.

Cloves are the flower buds of an evergreen tree of the myrtle family cultivated in the East and West Indies, Ceylon, Mauritius, Brazil, Guinea, and Sumatra. Spicy scented clove buds are highly prized in cookery, and provide an inexpensive way to scent soaps, perfumes, and incense.

Apply the mildly antiseptic oil of clove to infected teeth to relieve toothaches. The oil also cures athlete's foot and other fungal infections. Chew on clove buds to quell stomach gasses and eliminate halitosis.

Since clove buds are said to make a lover do one's bidding, it is a favorite ingredient of love potions. The buds also allegedly help nurture friendships, stop slander, and bring comfort and solace to one who has lost a loved one.

(RED) CLOVER
Names: *Trifolium pratense*, **Trefoil, Beebread, Cow Clover, Meadow Clover, Purple Clover.**
Associations: Jupiter, the Tuatha de Dannan of Irish mythology.

The red type does not attract bees as readily as the white variety (*T. repens*), but makes a good soil improving cover crop and fodder.

This alterative and antispasmodic is beneficial in cases of bronchial congestion and whooping cough. Powder the blossoms and make a poultice to attenuate the symptoms of cancer.

Clover is valuable in spells to attract business, money, and wealth, and is a prime ingredient of prosperity oil. Allegedly the blossoms chase away evil or alien spirits. A four-leafed clover is considered a good luck charm. The three- leafed clover symbolizes the Holy Trinity, and therefore, protection against evil.

COLTSFOOT
Names: *Tussilago farfara,* **Coughwort, Horsehoof, Son-before-the-father.**
Associations: Mercury, Venus.

Heart-shaped coltsfoot leaves (formed like a colt's foot) combined with mullein and other ingredients, substitutes for tobacco. Collect the leaves in June or July. Scottish country folk formerly stuffed pillows and mattresses with the silky hair tufts.

This herb enjoys a reputation as a demulcent, expectorant, emollient, anti-inflammatory, and tonic. Smoke the leaves or drink the tea in combination with horehound to cure a cough or bronchitis, or to relieve asthma. Unfortunately, coltsfoot has been linked with cancerous tumors of the liver, so the FDA discourages its internal use.

Coltsfoot leaves comprise an ingredient in spells for money, wealth, and general improvement of business prospects.

COMFREY
Names: *Symphytum officinale*, **Ass-ear, Bruisewort, Knitbone. This herb often is confused with boneset. The name in Latin means "to strengthen."**
Associations: Saturn, Capricorn.

It is now considered a poisonous plant by the FDA, which has performed some tests that show that comfrey can produce cancer in humans. However, it remains a popular botanical with herbalists. It thrives in the shade on damp ground, grows enormous leaves, and spreads readily. Comfrey contains protein and carotene, and thus can be consumed as a vegetable like spinach. It retains large amounts of vitamin B-12, and as such, may be used topically to facilitate new skin growth and to prevent wrinkles.

Comfrey is a demulcent, astringent, expectorant, hemostatic, vulnerary, expectorant, nutritive tonic, and alterative. It is a reputed blood purifier, and also is good for boils and other skin troubles. Herbalists recommend it be taken internally to alleviate gastric ulcers, eczema, asthma, tuberculosis, and rheumatism. This botanical mends broken bones and assuages the pain from cancerous swellings and nerve damage.

Comfrey leaves comprise an ingredient of business and wealth spells, and miscellaneous talismans. Place a few leaves in your baggage when travelling to assure an uneventful journey and safe arrival of your luggage.

CORIANDER

Names: *Coriandrum sativum,* **Cilantro.**
Associations: Mars, Moon.

The seeds of this common herb become quite fragrant when dried. It is used as a condiment in currys, soups, and Mexican-style dishes.

Herbalists tout the benefits of this botanical as an aromatic, carminative, active purgative, diuretic, alterative, stomachic, and stimulant. It is recommended to ease stomach aches, and when added to laxatives, prevents griping. Flavor medicine with coriander to disguise the bitter taste. Chewing too many seeds can have a narcotic effect.

Carry the seeds to insure good health and freedom from head-aches. The seeds allegedly help keep one's mate from wandering. Powdered seeds added to wine stimulate the passions. Coriander was considered one of the five sacred herbs that God required the Israelites to eat at Passover.

COUCH GRASS

Names: *Agropyron repens,* **Creeping Field-wheat, Dog Grass (because it is popular with the canine set as an emetic), Quack Grass, Witchgrass.**

Associations: Jupiter, Gemini.

This coarse perennial grass is used as a coffee substitute in emergency rations and as a cattle fodder because of its high carbohydrate content. For those who do not want to cultivate it, couch grass can be a troublesome weed in landscaped places, but the same rhizomes that make it tough to eradicate in lawns also prevent soil erosion in naturalized areas.

The diuretic beverage tea brewed from couch grass has a soothing effect on the urinary tract and alleviates cystitis.

It is considered a protection herb. Place a mojo bag filled with couch grass under your pillow during the times when you are performing other love spells to attract and keep the love of someone you admire from afar. Here is a spell to chase away feelings of discouragement and despair: "1/4 oz doggrass, 2 oz. yellow dock, 1 oz. khus khus. Mix thoroughly and sprinkle a pinch in each corner of every room of your home once every seven days."[12] In Black Magic, couch grass spread on the clay image of an enemy will kill or maim.

CUBEB
Name: *Piper cubeba*, Tailed Pepper.
Associations: Mercury, Mars.

Use the spicy berries of this climbing East Indian perennial plant in incense, medicine, and Magic. In coffee growing regions, it often is planted with the coffee trees so that the trees will shade and support the cubeb.

Cubeb is a stimulant, antiseptic, and carminative, beneficial for urethritis, prostate trouble, abscesses, piles, gonorrhea, catarrh, cystitis, and chronic bronchitis.

Carry the dried berries to bring good fortune, attract lovers, and keep evil spirits away. The Arabs, who introduced this peppery plant to the Western world, believed it to be an aphrodisiac. This is why in ancient times, people ate candy to which they added the powdered berries in order to cure them of frigidity. Add the berries to Hexbreaker incense to drive away demons.

DAMIANA
Name: *Turnera aphrodisiaca*.
Associations: Aphrodite, Iemanjá (Brazil), Pluto.

Damiana is a somewhat bitter-tasting botanical that grows as a shrub in the warmer climates of the Western hemisphere. The pale green, ribbed leaves with somewhat hairy undersides are the part of the plant that is used.

It is a diuretic, mild purgative, and tonic. Mrs. Grieve claims that it works directly on the reproductive organs to produce a stimulating, aphrodisiac effect.[13]

It is a vital ingredient of love potions and love charms. To attract good luck, wear a sachet filled with damiana leaves and anointed with verbena oil, and replace the leaves at every Quarter Moon.

DANDELION
Names: *Taraxacum officinale*, Dent-de-leon, Pissabed (named for its diuretic properties!), Priest's Crown (because the crown looks like a monk's bald pate after the flower drops its seeds), Swine's Snout (because of its resemblance after blooming to this part of a pig's anatomy).
Associations: Jupiter, Sun, Taurus, Sagittarius.

An ubiquitous plant common in most gardens, and in fact, almost impossible to eradicate. Dandelion has a milky root, notched leaves, and a cheery, yellow flower that attracts insects and bees. The roots may be roasted and ground with chicory as a coffee substitute. The tender leaves added to a spring salad provide ample amounts of vitamin C. The wine pressed from the blossoms is delicious.

It is a diuretic, hepatic tonic, astringent, stomachic, lithotropic, galactogogue, and cholagogue. It stimulates excretion of urine to help cure urinary and kidney infections. The vitamin C content benefits cases of scurvy and eczema.

Plant dandelion outside the northwest corner of your house to bring prosperity to all who live under your roof. Wear the flowers in a red charm bag sewn shut with white thread tied around your neck in order to make your wishes come true. Make a sachet of the leaves and rose petals, and scent it with lily-of- the-valley to overcome emotional pain.

To contact spirits on the astral plane, drink a cup of dandelion tea before retiring. Then refill your mug with more steaming brew and place it at your bedside.

DEER'S TONGUE

Names: *Trilisa odoratissima,* Hart's Tongue, Wild Vanilla, Vanilla Leaf.
Association: Damballah (Voodoo).

The leaves of this perennial herb native to North America, when dried, are added to incense and potpourris to impart a vanilla-like odor. Similarly, the leaves scent tobacco. The leaves are a demulcent, diaphoretic, and febrifuge.

In Voodoo, this is an offertory herb to Damballah. Hide a sachet of the leaves under the pillow of the person you desire to reveal secrets to you. If a man wraps deer's tongue leaves in a silk cloth and then goes to visit his girlfriend, she will be favorably disposed to his suggestions.

DILL

Name: *Anethum graveolens.*
Association: Mercury.

A hardy annual of the carrot family with umbrella-like flowers, this common kitchen garden herb flavors fish, pickles, chicken, breads, and cakes. The name originates with the Old Norse term, *dilla,* meaning "to lull." Dill is the "anise" of the Bible.

It is an aromatic, carminative, stimulant, and stomachic. In the old days it was believed that dill oil placed on a sugar cube and ingested was a panacea for children's complaints. People also ate it to lose weight.

All parts of the plant counteract Black Magic. The seeds boiled in wine are considered an aphrodisiac and brain stimulant. Carry the seeds for protection against negative Witchcraft. German brides of the fourteenth century tucked dill into their wedding bouquets to insure a happy marriage.

DRAGON'S BLOOD

Names: *Daemonorops draco, Dracaena draco.*
Associations: Mars, Aries, Pluto, Gemini.

Dragon's blood consists of a red resin exuded from the fruit of a kind of palm tree native to Sumatra and Borneo. It is used commercially to color varnishes and tinctures. The best quality is wrapped in a palm leaf while still soft, and exported.

However, the palm-leafed wrapped resin has become exceedingly difficult to obtain, and only chunks or powder seem to be available through botanical suppliers. Some herbalists believe that dragon's blood possibly cures diarrhea and syphilis.

Magically, it is used in charms for wealth, health, and love. Carry chunks of the resin to cure impotence and bring good fortune in love, business, money matters, and gambling. At the beginning of a ritual, trace with the powder the symbol of the pentagram, or any other protective sign to insulate the Circle.

Make dragon's blood ink by dissolving the powder in alcohol. Trace your magical sigils and inscriptive talismans with the ink, but take care: a little powder goes a long way. So I discovered when I once added too much to a protection bath salt I was experimenting with. I walked around looking like Rudolph the Red-Nosed Reindeer for days!

ELECAMPANE

Names: *Inula helenium*, Helen's Flower (because according to Greek mythology, the flower sprang from the tears of Helen of Troy), Scabwort, Elf Dock, Wild Sunflower, Horseheal.
Associations: Sun, Mercury, Jupiter.

This member of the aster family is a tall, hardy perennial with bright yellow flowers that resemble sunflowers, but are violet scented. The root is used in medicine. Distill the green leaves as a wash or facial steam to make your complexion clear and fair.

A diuretic, alterative, astringent (particularly in veterinary medicine), diaphoretic, expectorant, stomachic, stimulant, cholagogue, and possible antibiotic. It soothes coughs and other pulmonary complaints and skin diseases.

Elecampane comprises an ingredient of love potions because of its alleged aphrodisiac and restorative effects. Ancient peoples carried a handful when travelling through the forest or desert to protect them against the bites and stings of poisonous insects and snakes. The scent from the dried herb is alleged to calm the savage breast.

EYEBRIGHT

Names: *Euphrasia officinalis*. Meadow Eyebright, Red Eyebright.
Associations: Sun; of the Three Graces, eyebright is associated with the one who represents joy and mirth.

Mrs. Grieve calls this an "elegant little plant" of the snapdragon family.[14] More than twenty species exist. It is a delicate, semi-parasitic botanical with tiny two- and three-lobed white or red flowers. Because it takes nutrition from the roots of other plants, I advise you to grow it in a grassy area to take advantage of its extensive root system.

An alterative, anti-inflammatory, astringent, and tonic, it is taken internally and in an eyewash to cure eye diseases such as conjunctivitis (in combination with golden seal). Homeopathic doses are said to withstand scrofula. Smoke the leaves to ameliorate chronic bronchial pain.

Drink the tea along with queen-of-the-meadow and sage to enhance psychic visions and to produce clarity of vision when you wish to concentrate the force of your will toward a specific purpose. In *Paradise Lost,* the Archangel Michael rubs Adam's eyes with eyebright to enable him to see the future mortality of men.

FENNEL
Names: *Foeniculum vulgare,* **Sweet Fennel, Wild Fennel.**
Associations: Mercury, Virgo, Diana, Jupiter.

An umbelliferous plant similar to dill and anise in appearance, taste, and medicinal action, fennel flavors soups, salads, and fish. It is also an antispasmodic, diuretic, expectorant, galactogogue, stimulant, mild carminative, and purgative. If you are dieting, you can chew fennel to suppress your appetite. It eases stomach aches and promotes digestion. Administer it with eyebright in an eyewash.

Carry this botanical in your pocket or purse along with St. John's-wort to ward off negative Witchcraft. In medieval times people believed that if they blocked their keyholes with fennel, the herb would discourage ghosts from entering the house. Alternatively, you may hang this botanical over your doorway to protect your home. The ancients thought that by consuming fennel they gained strength, courage, and longevity. In the language of flowers this herb signifies "strength."

FEVERFEW
Names: *Chrysanthemum parthenium,* **Bachelor's-button, Featherfew, Featherfoil, Wild Chamomile.**
Associations: Venus, Sagittarius.

The flowers resemble the flowers of Roman chamomile. This plant grows upright approximately 2 1/2-feet tall. It is used as an insect repellant, particularly to keep away bees. Plant some around your house to purify the air. In cooking, feverfew is used to flavor pastries, fried eggs, and wines.

It is reputed to break fevers, promote menstruation, and treat female problems. A tincture used as a balm alleviates the pain from bee stings. In former times, feverfew was used to treat nervousness, hysteria, low spirits, colds, indigestion, and diarrhea.

Carry a red mojo bag sachet of feverfew flowers when travelling, visiting hospitals, or engaging in dangerous sports or work, as it will help defend you against accidents and illness. Drink the tea during stressful times as a relaxant and to strengthen your system against illness.

FLAX

Names: *Linum usitatissimum*, Linseed, Lint Bells.
Associations: Mercury, Gemini.

The fibers from this blue-flowered plant have been used to weave linens for 10,000 years. The oil pressed from the seeds is used in oilcloth, paints, varnishes, and linoleums.

The seeds of this demulcent and laxative are a natural mucilage. Grind them into poultices and apply to burns and boils, and as an ingredient in cough syrup. Flax is also effective against constipation and urinary tract infections.

Because flax makes a very white linen, it became a symbol of purity in ancient Egypt. It was used to weave the pharaohs' shrouds, and, later, robes for the priests of the Hebrews and Greeks. Flax protects against negative Witchcraft. Keep the seeds in a dish in the living room to purify the atmosphere and drive away disruptive influences.

FRANKINCENSE

Names: *Boswellia thurifera, B. carterii*, Olibanum.
Associations: Sun, Apollo, Sagittarius, Leo, Aquarius.

A free-burning gum resin from the inner wood of a deciduous tree, frankincense is employed mainly in incense-making. The tree grows in Africa and the Arab countries.

Its medicinal action is mainly a stimulant. In the old days, frankincense was a cure for bronchitis and laryngitis, and was particularly valued as a steam inhalant and cure for genito-urinary tract infections and leprosy. However, it has fallen into disuse as a remedy during this century. Combine the powder with beaten egg whites for a fine facial tonic.

As the legend goes, an ancient Persian king buried alive his daughter, Leucothea, to keep Apollo from winning her affections. Apollo sprinkled nectar and ambrosia on her grave, which seeped into her corpse and blossomed forth as the frankincense tree.

Frankincense was an offertory herb and incense of the Egyptians, Babylonians, and Jews. The Hebrews stored the precious commodity in a great chamber of the house of god in Jerusalem. The Egyptians also charred the resin to a black powder in order to paint their eyelids.

GALANGAL

Names: *Alpinia officinarum* **(the name is an Arabic corruption of a Chinese term which means "mild ginger"), Galanga, Catarrh Root. Associations: Aries, the Exus and Pombas-Giras of Brazilian folk religion.**

The rhizome is the part used. It has a pungent spicy taste, and is an aromatic in incense-making and tea. This carminative, stimulant, and antipyretic relieves flatulence, dyspepsia, seasickness, and vomiting.

In medieval times galangal was valued as an aphrodisiac. Carry the rhizome into court to influence a verdict in your favor, or secrete it in your pocket or purse when seeking employment.

GARLIC

Names: *Allium sativum*, **Poor-man's Treacle.**
Associations: Mars, Aries.

It may come as a surprise to learn that this plant with long, flat, pointed leaves, topped with pinkish-white flowers and with an extremely odiferous bulb composed of pungent cloves is actually a member of the lily family. Garlic is famous throughout the world for the strong, but irresistible flavor it imparts to many ethnic dishes.

An antiseptic, antispasmodic, diuretic, and expectorant, this botanical is healthy for the body. It is used to help cure colds, coughs, sore throats, intestinal disorders, intestinal worms, rheumatism, and snakebite. It has been proven to lower blood pressure and blood cholesterol levels. The cloves are chock full of vitamins such as A, B-1 (thiamine), B-2 (riboflavin), and C.

The ancients extolled the physical and psychical benefits of garlic, and believed it granted them strength and courage. Thus, the pyramid builders consumed it as well as the soldiers of the Roman legions.

This botanical is renowned from ancient to modern times as a charm against evil, especially vampires (as is attested amply by Hollywood vampire movies), ghosts, poltergeists, and the plague. It is perfectly possible that at least in the latter case, there might be some truth to the myth, as fleas tend to shun garlic-exuding skin for tastier meals. In modern times garlic is used in spells to clear the mind and render a person better able to make choices and judgments.

An old Voodoo spell to prevent a person from being crossed requires you to bathe in a tub full of warm water to which you have added 1 teaspoon each of garlic, basil, sage and parsley, 1/4 teaspoon saltpeter, and 1/2 teaspoon geranium water. Bathe in the potion every Monday, Wednesday and Friday until you feel the danger has passed. On leaving the bath, rub your body with bay rum, and anoint yourself with verbena and honeysuckle oils. At least the perfume oils will help neutralize the pungent garlicky odor.

GENTIAN
Names: *Gentania villosa, G. lutea, G. acaulis,* Marsh Gentian, Pale Gentian, Striped Gentian, Sampson's Snakeroot. The plant is named for Gentius, a second-century B.C. king of Illyria, who allegedly discovered its medicinal uses.
Associations: Mars, Aries, Mercury.

This plant of over 180 species usually grows in the semi-shaded dry areas of meadows and woodlands. It is an eighteen-inch tall perennial, native to North America. The funnel-like, greenish-white to purplish-green flowers and lanced to oval-shaped leaves are its most distinctive features.

Many ancient medicinal uses for this plant have been recorded on Egyptian papyrus, including remedies against snakebite, gout, rabies, and rheumatism. It is ingested to stimulate the appetite.

The folk of Appalachia believe that if they carry a root in their pockets, it increases their physical strength. Add an infusion of gentian root and dragon's blood bath crystals to your bath water to attract friends. Keep the powdered root in an envelope in your pocket or wallet to keep thieves away.

GINGER
Names: *Zingiber officinale,* Roscoe.
Associations: Sun, Mars, Moon.

The aromatic, silvery-brown rootstalk of this tropical perennial is a zesty culinary spice. The fragrant blue and yellow flowers that bloom at the top of a pointed spike blend well in perfumery. Ginger is a spicy component of Rising Moon anointing oil.

The root is a diaphoretic, carminative, stimulant, rubefacient, and emmenagogue. It is beneficial for dyspepsia, flatulent colic, diarrhea, and chest complaints. Suck on candied ginger to help overcome motion sickness.

Offer whole wild ginger root to the elemental spirits, especially at the Eight Great Sabbats. Like many spicy herbs, ginger is considered an aphrodisiac, particularly adept at curing frigidity.

In *The Modern Witch's Spellbook vol. II,*[15] Sarah Morrison suggests that if you see someone you would like to get to know at the grocery store, you should manage to drop a piece of ginger root in the person's shopping basket, and she/he will follow you to the checkout. After that, it's up to you!

GOLDENSEAL
Names: *Hydrastis canadensis,* Indian Paint, Yellow Root, Yellow Puccoon, Eyeroot, Ground Raspberry.
Associations: Sun, the gods of the Cherokee Indians, Venus.

Goldenseal is an important North American Indian wildflower, and member of the buttercup family. The fruit resembles a raspberry, but is not edible. The root yields a brilliant yellow dye.

A stomachic, laxative, alterative, antiseptic, diuretic, and powerful hemostatic, the herb is poisonous if consumed in large doses; so I recommend you prescribe it with care. If taken in very small doses it alleviates morning sickness (large doses will make a pregnant woman miscarry), vomiting, eczema, eye inflammations, and liver diseases.

If you own a store and would like to attract customers, sprinkle a pinch of golden seal in each corner of the shop every morning, and watch your business grow!

HEART'S-EASE

Names: *Viola tricolor,* **Pansy (from the French word** *pensée,* **meaning "thought"), Johnny-jump-up, Ladies' Delight. The flower receives its name from the belief that its scent soothes the emotions of unhappy lovers.**
Associations: Saturn, Libra.

Heart's-ease is a common, fifteen-inch tall annual that throws so many seeds it easily resows itself. Its common habitat is at the edge of the forest, and semi-shaded woods. From my gardening experience, I have found that if you mulch the plants they will winter over. The tri-colored flowers are purple, white, and yellow. The more fragrant variety is called *V. odorata.*

This botanical is a diuretic, expectorant, demulcent, and laxative. The flowers are the part used as a blood purifier, sedative, and external remedy for itching, scabs, and ulcers.

The flowers are an ingredient of love potions. Put them in your shoes to attract a lover.

HEATHER

Names: *Calluna vulgaris,* **Scotch Heather, Hall.**
Association: Venus

The wiry stems of this shrubby evergreen that grows on barren, sandy, or rocky heaths in Scotland have been used for centuries to make brooms and thatching for roofs. The tops and flowers are boiled to render a subtle, yellow dye. The flowers also produce a brownish colored honey that is thought to be an ingredient of Drambuie. The plant is an antitussive, diuretic, and sedative.

White heather enjoys a reputation as a good luck charm, and as such, is tucked into bridal bouquets. In times gone by, people burned heather in rainmaking spells. Witches were supposed to ride to their Sabbats on heather brooms.

BLACK HELLEBORE

Names: *Helleborus niger,* **Christmas Rose, Melampode. The** *Veratrum viride* **plant which is sometimes called Hellebore, is also known as Indian Poke Root.**
Association: Saturn.

This highly poisonous plant is a perennial that blossoms red or white in the winter. The dropped blossoms and leaves from this popular, colorful Christmas-flowering houseplant have been known to poison pets.

Not for internal consumption, but traditionally, it was used as a drastic purgative and for cases of dropsy and amenorrhea. The root of the hellebore plant is a violent irritant and should be avoided.

French sorcerers believed that to carry the root made them invincible. Cattle were blessed with the root to keep them immune to illness, accidents, and other evils.

HIBISCUS
Names: *Hibiscus rosa-sinensis*, China Rose, Chinese Hibiscus, Hawaiian Hibiscus, Rose-of-China.
Association: Venus.

Over 300 species of this lovely flowering evergreen shrub- tree are known. The red or orange petals are used to flavor tea and also produce a black dye for shoes, hair, and eyebrows. The flowers are an astringent and also used in potpourri to add purple highlights. The root is a demulcent that soothes the respiratory and digestive system. The bark is reputed to regulate the menstrual cycle.

In the language of flowers, this plant stands for "delicate beauty." Use it in love potions.

HOPS
Names: *Humulus lupulus.* The English name derives from an Anglo-Saxon term meaning "to climb."
Associations: Mars, Sun, Pluto.

Hops is a climbing, perennial vine of the hemp family, commonly found in wastelands of countries in the northern temperate zone. The greenish-pink, fruity cones resemble clover flowers.

Over time, hops has fulfilled many useful purposes in wortcunning. The leaves and flowers make a brown dye, the flowers have been used to brew beer since the fourteenth century. A type of paper called "bine" formerly was made from the stem. The Romans even ate the young spring shoots, which taste much like asparagus.

The flowers are recommended as a nervine, diuretic, sedative, tonic, galactogogue, anodyne, and preservative. An infusion helps calm nervous disorders and induces sleep. Hops promotes a good appetite and quells indigestion. It counteracts jaundice, bladder, stomach, and liver disorders. Administer it externally with poppy heads to reduce the inflammation and pain associated with neuralgia.

Before its beer-brewing value was appreciated, hops was thought to breed melancholy. Stuff this botanical into a sleep pillow with chamomile and rosemary to prevent nightmares and nocturnal attacks on the astral plane. It also brings a restful sleep to babies. Inexplicably, at least to me, in the language of plants, this botanical stands for "injustice."

HOREHOUND

Names: *Marrubium vulgare,* Hoar-hound, White Horehound, Marvel.
Associations: Mercury, Scorpio.

This wooly leafed herb of the mint family has toothed, wrinkled leaves that grow on whitish-gray, woody, square stems. Horehound was a favorite flavoring used by American settlers as an ingredient in candy and cough drops. This expectorant, laxative, and sedative is an appetite stimulant used in bitters. Syrup made from the leaves soothes sore throats. The ancient Greeks administered horehound to treat female infertility.

Mix horehound and ash leaves in a bowl of water and place it by the inside of your bedroom door at night to keep evil spirits from entering. Don't forget to throw out the water in the morning and renew nightly until the danger has passed.

HYSSOP

Names: *Hyssopus officinalis,* Holy Herb.
Associations: Moon, Mars, Jupiter, Cancer.

A bushy, highly aromatic herb of the mint family, hyssop displays blue flowers and narrow, pointed leaves. Grow it in your vegetable garden to discourage cabbage butterflies.

It is a vulnerary, expectorant (flowers), carminative, diaphoretic, and stimulant. An infusion of the leaves remedies asthma, loosens phlegm, and soothes sore throats. The ancients applied hyssop to infections caused by wounds to warriors, and to restore torn tissue. Later it was discovered that the leaves contain penicillin.

As a symbol of purification, strew hyssop around the ritual Circle or place a bowlful on the altar. Dip a hyssop sprig into Holy Water to purify the coveners as they enter the Circle. Rub it on a mirror in a candlelit room, and sit in meditation to obtain psychic visions.

IRISH MOSS

Names: *Chondrus crispus,* **Carrageen.**
Associations: Jupiter, Neptune, Pisces, Morgan.

Irish moss is a type of yellow, green, red or purple seaweed found on beaches along the North Atlantic coast. It is an emulsifier in facial and body creams, and a nutritive herb eaten to stave off hunger pangs in times of famine.

This unimpressive looking seaweed is prized as a demulcent, emollient, laxative, nutritive, and excellent remedy for pulmonary, kidney and bladder disorders. For a tasty, nutritive tonic combine one-half ounce of the botanical with an equal amount of cocoa, and boil the mixture in three pints of milk for ten to fifteen minutes. Strain and season with licorice or cinnamon, and sweeten with honey.

Place the dried weed under your carpets to attract good luck to your home.

JALAP

Names: *Ipomaea purga,* **Bindweed, High John the Conqueror Root.**
The common name is derived from the city of Xalapa, Mexico, near where this climbing plant flourishes in the wild.
Associations: Mars, Aries.

This elegant, twining plant with pink to crimson flowers grows in Mexico and South America. It is prized for its spike-shaped root. Since the root contains prussic acid and is a strong cathartic and purgative, I do not recommend it for medicinal use. However, traditionally it has been applied in extreme cases of constipation and intestinal worms.

Jalap, or John the conqueror root, is one of the most popular talismanic roots in Witchcraft. It seems to be something of an occult panacea. For example, it is alleged to attract love, prosperity, success against all odds, and victory in court. Moreover, it is held to neutralize melancholy, bad moods, confusion of thought, and evil spirits. In Voodoo, a popular gris-gris to attract a woman to a man entails soaking the root in sugar water for twenty-four hours before wrapping it in a conjure bag.

KAVA KAVA

Names: *Piper methysticum,* **Intoxicating Pepper.**
Associations: Scorpio, Pluto.

The pungent, aromatic root of this shrub native to Australia and Polynesia is the part used. The leaves are large, webbed, and heart-shaped.

This diuretic, tonic, nervine, analgesic, antiseptic and sedative counteracts insomnia, heals vaginitis, genito-urinary tract infections, and gonorrhea. The chewed root is a narcotic and stimulant. Ingested in large, regular doses, kava-kava can cause toxic substances to accumulate in the liver.

Because of this botanical's highly regarded aphrodisiac properties, it is an ingredient much sought for love potions. Chew, or drink the chopped root as a beverage tea before retiring to cause clear, easily remembered, epic-length dreams.

KELP
Names: *Laminaria digitata,* **Tangleweed;** *L. saccharina,* **Sugar Wrack.**
Associations: Neptune, Pisces.

Kelp is a generic name for any of a number of large, brown seaweeds visible only at low tide. They are rich in vitamins A, B, B-2, B-3, B-12, C, E, K, aluminum, barium, bismith, boron, calcium, chlorine, chromium, cobalt, copper, gallium, iodine, magnesium, manganese, molybdenum, phosphorus, sodium, potassium, selenium, sulphur, and zinc. Kelp makes a nutritious crop fertilizer and condiment for soup, salads, and meats. It is used in the production of iodine and as a stabilizing agent in many packaged foods.

This botanical is so valued among herbalists for its vitamin content that it has earned a reputation as a "brain food." It cleanses arteries and the reproductive system, increases vitality, and remedies eczema, asthma, anemia, headache, goiter, and rickets.

Marie Laveau, the Voodoo queen, recommended that to insure a full congregation at Church, the minister should wash the floor with a gallon of water that has been steeped for seven days with one teaspoonful of kelp, one teaspoonful of nutmeg, and a pinch of orris powder.

LADY'S MANTLE
Names: *Alchemilla vulgaris,* **Bear's-foot, Lion's-foot, Nine Hooks.**
The Latin name links this botanical to Alchemy — a tribute to the high repute in which it once was held. Alchemists have attempted

to distill essence of lady's mantle to discover the secret of eternal youth.

Associations: Venus, Sun.

The hooked leaves of this elegant member of the rose family are pleated like a lady's cloak of former times. Clusters of small, yellowish-green flowers bloom from July to August.

A hemostatic, tonic, astringent, and vulnerary, lady's mantle heals ruptures and strengthens muscles, draws water from the kidneys, and regularizes the shape of the womb after childbirth.

Teas brewed with lady's mantle and horehound, and consumed daily are alleged to increase female fertility. It is thought to bring untroubled sleep if placed under the pillow.

Because the leaf folds up like an umbrella and retains a drop of morning dew, the entrapped dew was likened to the essence of the womb, and was prized by Alchemists.

A sachet of this botanical is said to confer self-control, dignity, and distinction.

LADY'S SLIPPER

Names: *Cypripedium pubescens, C. parviflorum, C, calceolus,* **American Valerian, Noah's Ark, Moccasin Flower, Yellow Indian Shoe, Nerveroot.**

Associations: Venus, the Great Goddess, Gemini.

This perennial orchid that grows in forests has a yellow, moccasin-like flower and eight-inch oval leaves. The root of the orchid is a nervine, antispasmodic, slight psychedelic, sedative, and gentle nervous stimulant, less powerful than valerian. It relieves headaches and checks epilepsy.

Lady's slipper makes an appropriate offering to place at waterfalls and forest henges (sacred places made in the forest) to honor the goddess. In the language of flowers, the plant symbolizes "fickleness."

LAVENDER

Names: *Lavandula vera* **(English lavender),** *L . officinalis, L. spica.* **The word derives from** *lavare,* **Latin for "to wash." Romans loved washing in lavender oil because of its clean, fresh scent.**

Associations: Mercury, Jupiter, Sun.

A generally shrubby, perennial plant of the mint family, it will winter over in cold climates if carefully mulched. The French and Spanish varieties do not, in my opinion, produce as superior quality oil as the true English variety. English lavender is cultivated in quantity now only in the lavender fields of Norfolk, England.

It has been used since Roman times in perfumery to scent apparel, leather, linens, etc., and to embalm bodies. It once was the custom to scent a bride's bedclothes with lavender on her wedding night because the fragrance was thought to soothe her fears. It also makes a refreshing and attractive edible garnish.

The flowers are an antispasmodic and expectorant. Gargle an infusion to cure a hoarse voice. Use this botanical also as an insect repellent or to relieve headaches and intestinal gas.

Lavender is an ingredient of psychic dream pillows. In Iberia on St. John's Day, peasants used to build bonfires, which they stoked with lavender sprigs to purify the area and cause evil spirits to flee.

French lavender is one ingredient of Four Thieves Vinegar, which fulfills various magical purposes in Voodoo. Add lavender to money spells to give them vigor.

This herb also is used in spells with couch grass, wood betony and violet leaves to promote peace and happiness in the home. Some occultists claim lavender helps assuage feelings of unresolved guilt. Nevertheless, in the language of flowers, the plant symbolizes "destruction."

LEMON BALM
Names: *Melissa officinalis,* Melissa, Sweet Balm, Balm.
Associations: Sun, Jupiter, Cancer.

It is a bushy, lemon-scented plant of the mint family with delicate, white flowers that grows one-to-three feet high, and attracts bees to the garden. It is grown widely in Europe, Asia, and America, and is a favorite in herb gardens. The leaves make a delicious beverage tea, both hot and iced.

This botanical is regarded as a diaphoretic, antispasmodic, antipyretic, emmenagogue, sedative, tonic, and gentle stimulant. It is beneficial in cases of hysteria, stomach cramps, irregular menses, poor digestion, and colic. The herb seems to alleviate nausea, sore throat, aching teeth, and soothe the pain of bee stings.

Miguel Tierra says it neutralizes diseases which arise from being in situations that a person is not ready to accept.[16]

Lemon balm comprises an essential ingredient of love potions, and is particularly potent when added to bath water. Steep the leaves in wine and drink the brew to chase away melancholy and rejuvenate yourself.

Anoint your third eye with the oil to receive answers to questions and to predict future events, or anoint your upper lip and palms of your hands with lemon balm before speaking in public or writing so that your audience will pay heed.

LICORICE
Names: *Glycyrrhiza glabra, G. lepidota,* American Licorice. The origin of the name is a Greek word meaning "sweet root."
Associations: Mercury, Gemini.

The root of this feathery plant is fifty times sweeter than sugar. It is a multi-talented botanical: after extracting the sweetness from the root, the residuals can be used to make a foam for fire extinguishers; a fertilizer is derived from it; the root also flavors ice cream, beer and ale, and masks the bitter taste of medicines; the powder is added to some pills to stiffen the pill mass and prevent them from adhering to each other; it is a safe sweetener for diabetics.

Fourteen species comprise the genus, but most of them will not stand a severe frost. The plant is found in sandy soil near stream beds. Other than its susceptibility to frost, it is a hardy plant, little subject to the ravages of pests and disease. Research currently is being carried out in Britain to isolate certain chemicals contained in licorice as a possible AIDS preventative.

Herbalists make claims for licorice as a demulcent, blood purifier, expectorant, laxative, and alterative. Because it contains substances similar to adrenal cortical hormones, it is administered to treat adrenal disorders. Licorice suppresses coughs, colds, stomach and intestinal troubles, ulcers, stress-related disorders, and hoarseness. As an alterative, it normalizes the female hormonal balance. It is said to promote fertility in both males and females.

Alexander the Great distributed licorice to his soldiers because he believed that this sacred plant would protect them and make them strong. King Tut carried the root with him to the grave to ease his journey to the Otherworld. Use it in spells to arouse the passions of a loved one, gain power over another, or to change a person's mind.

LIFE EVERLASTING
Names: *Gnaphaliam genus,* **American Everlasting, Cudweed.**
Association: Leo.

Use the lanceate leaves and downy stalks medicinally. The dried flowers are a lovely, yellow color, and although odorless, make an attractive ingredient for potpourris and dried flower arrangements.

This anodyne, astringent, and pectoral counteracts diarrhea, dysentery, and bronchitis. In a poultice it eases the pain from bruises, sprains, boils, and swellings.

As the name indicates, it is believed that a person can imbibe a daily cup of life everlasting tea for a prolonged and healthy life. Or fulfill the same wish by keeping some dried flowers in a closet or in a drawer.

LOBELIA
Names: *Lobelia inflata, L. cardinalis* **(red-flowered variety known as Red Cardinal), Indian Tobacco, Asthma Weed, Pukeweed, Bladderpod, Vomitroot, Gagroot.**
Associations: Jupiter, Neptune.

Named after Matthias de Lobel, physician and botanist to James I, lobelia is found throughout the dry, northern regions of the United States and Canada. The erect, hairy stems grow oval, serrated leaves, and tiny blue or lavender flowers that transform into green fruit. Use the leaves and seeds.

Lobelia can be lethal if ingested in large doses; so prescribe with care. An antiasthmatic, diaphoretic, euphoriant, expectorant, nervine, emetic, and sedative, the herb has been used traditionally to relieve asthma, convulsions, epilepsy, inflammations, diptheria, and tonsilitis. Smoke the dried leaves to curb the desire for tobacco. Note, however, that this plant is considered poisonous by the FDA.

In the language of flowers, lobelia means "malevolence."

LOTUS
Name: *Nymphaea genus.*
Associations: Isis, Hathor, Thoth, Neptune, Ra.

The lotus is a lovely water lily whose beauty has made it a familiar subject for Oriental painters.

An infusion of root makes an effective vaginal douche, and it is chopped up and eaten in Oriental cuisine.

Lotus is sacred to the great religions of India, Tibet, China, and Egypt, as well as to the Qabalists. An ancient Greek legend tells how it was eaten by the Lotophagi to induce forgetfulness and a dreamlike state. Among other associations, the flower stands for beauty, power of mind over matter, and chastity.

The root is a love talisman. Use it in rituals to invoke the ancient Egyptian deities, or fashion it into a pendulum to divine the future. Another way to scry with the root is to carve or write "yes" on one side and "no" on the other, and toss it into the air to see which side lands up.

LOVAGE
Names: *Levisticum officinale,* Italian Lovage, Garden Lovage, *Ligusticum scotium* (Scotch Lovage, a related plant), Sea Parsley. Associations: Taurus, Sun.

A favorite, tall perennial in old English herb gardens, the leaves, root and fruit are highly aromatic, smelling a bit like celery. Blanched, the stems are eaten like celery. Lovage also makes a delicious tea, similar in flavor to angelica. Add it to facials to help smooth away wrinkles.

This antipyretic, aromatic, carminative, diuretic, emmenagogue, and stimulant also contains large amounts of vitamin C; so it effectively treats deficiency of this vitamin. The plant cures urinary ailments, colic, flatulence, and halitosis.

Lovage is a component of money spells. Carry it to attract customers to stores and increase your popularity and good luck. If suspended in a mojo bag from a silk thread and worn around the neck next to the skin, it is alleged to attract a lover and enhance one's psychic abilities.

MAIDENHAIR
Names: *Adiantum capillus, A. veneris,* Hair of Venus, Rock Fern. Associations: Venus, Mercury.

When a branch of this dainty fern is immersed in water, it appears silvery, and when retrieved from the water, it remains dry. The plant grows in moist caves and on rocks near the sea, on damp walls, and on the sides of wells.

It is beneficial to asthma. Swallow it in a syrup to mitigate pulmonary catarrhs.

For centuries, the common folk have believed in the beautifying powers of the maidenhair fern, and held that to carry it enhanced a person's natural beauty. In the language of flowers, it means "discretion."

MARIGOLD

Names: *Calendula officinalis,* **Pot Marigold. The origin of the name is probably "gold of the Virgin Mary."**
Association: Sun.

Prized for its bright flowers, which range in color from white to yellow, orange, and deep red, this hardy annual is easy to grow from seed, and provides an edible garnish. It has been used to color cheese, cloth, and hair. Plant marigolds as a border in your vegetable garden to discourage pests and to draw solar energy.

Only the leaves and flower of the common orange variety possess any medicinal value. Prepare it in an ointment to heal wounds, sores, and inflammations.

The tea strengthens the heart, liver, and kidneys, eases menstrual tension, and expels toxins. It is a remedy for headache, toothache, flu, red eyes, and jaundice. Marigold tea also will draw out the rash of smallpox and measles.

Sew marigold flowers into sleep pillows to encourage psychic visions. Carry it into court to help win a case. Wear a sachet of marigold flowers when you wish to discover the identity of one who has robbed you. The flower petals strewn under your bed will make your dreams come true.

Added to the bath water, marigolds will help you win the respect of others. Combine the oil with thyme and meadowsweet oil, and anoint your forehead with it to see fairies. Plant marigolds at the front of your house to let the bounty of the Sun stream in.

MARJORAM / OREGANO

Names: *Origanum hortensis, O. marjorana,* **Sweet, or Pot Marjoram;**
O. vulgare, **Medicinal, or Wild Marjoram;** *O. heracleoticum,*
Oregano or Greek Oregano. In Greek *orbs* **and** *ganos* **combine to
mean "joy of the mountain."**
Associations: Venus, Mercury, Aries.

Marjoram is a common, tall perennial kitchen garden herb with
purple flowers used to flavor meats and beer. It combines well with
thyme. This herb also scents linens and potpourris. The tops make a
reddish-brown dye.

The slightly indented leaves are an antispasmodic, diaphoretic,
carminative, emmenagogue, expectorant, stomachic, and aromatic.
Marjoram cures nervous headaches. Apply an infusion of the leaves
externally to sprains and rheumatism. The plant's aroma quells
seasickness.

Oregano was said to be created by the gods of Mt. Olympus. In
Greece and Rome it was offered to the goddess of the hearth fire. It is
still a component of Vesta Fire incense. Use it in money spells, or
when performing a ritual to make financial gain through travel.

It is also a protective herb that prevents injury from lightning. The
Egyptians ate some each morning before leaving their beds to protect
them during the day. In days of old it was believed that thyme and
marjoram kept milk from curdling during a thunderstorm.

Add the dried leaves to charm bags to protect yourself against
negative Witchcraft, or plant it on a loved one's grave to insure a
happy afterlife.

Steep marjoram, marigold, thyme, and meadowsweet in mineral
oil for seven days. Strain the oil through cloth, and anoint your
forehead with it to communicate with the elemental spirits. Consecrate Mercury talismans with marjoram oil.

A fifteenth-century love charm calls for a blend of marjoram,
thyme, and honey, which girls ate to dream of their future husbands.
A combination of oregano, salt and white pepper is used in spells to
reveal the evil intentions of others. If you wish to attract a lifelong
mate, tack marjoram sprigs into the corners of your room. Renew
monthly.

MARSHMALLOW

Names: *Althaea officinalis* (the official name in Greek means "to heal"), Althea Root, Mallows, Mortification Root (so named because a poultice of the root prevents infections), Sweetweed (because it is used in candy making).
Associations: Moon, Venus.

The soft, downy, petiole leaves of this marsh plant grow on three- to four-foot stems in damp meadows and ditches. As an anti-inflammatory and demulcent, the mucilage from the root soothes skin and mucous membranes. An extract from the boiled plant placates sore throats and internal, and external inflammations.

Emperor Charlemagne held the marshmallow in such high esteem that he ordered it to be cultivated on his lands. It is an ingredient of Egyptian Papyrus, a special incense designed to call upon the Xu, elemental spirits of the Egyptian pantheon. To protect your child from harm, add this botanical to your baby's bath water.

Albertus Magnus thought that a combination of marshmallow, hollyhock, alum, and brimstone would enable a person to pass through fire without being burned.

MISTLETOE

Names: *Phorandendron flavescens* (American), *Viscum album* (European), Golden Bough.
Associations: Sun, Moon, Jupiter, Thor, the Druids.

Mistletoe is a scrubby parasite that grows on some trees, particularly the apple. Contrary to popular belief, it is seldom found on oaks. Because of its rare appearance on the oak, which in turn, was linked to the thunder god, mistletoe came to symbolize Mars-like attributes. Its golden color also is associated the Sun god.

It is a poisonous plant, particularly the berries. Although the flowers are open from February through April, the white berries do not ripen until winter.

As it is poisonous, I do not recommend medicinal use. However, the Druids believed the plant held the power to perform miraculous cures in almost any area of medicine. This is the probable origin of the custom of kissing under the mistletoe. It was credited especially with increasing human fertility and curing epilepsy.

Strew the cut herb around the Circle for protection. Make the sign of the cross surrounded by a Circle on your enemy's doorstep, and that person will surely never bother you again.

Mistletoe is a symbol of greeting, good will, and love. Balder the Beautiful, son of Odin, was killed by a mistletoe arrow. Later, when he was restored to life, Odin gave the mistletoe to the goddess of love for safekeeping; hence the present-day association of the plant with love.

MOTHERWORT

Names: *Leonurus cardiaca*, **Lion's-ear, Lion's-tail, Lion's-tart, Throwwort.**
Associations: Venus, Leo.

A plant of the mint family, motherwort grows in vacant lots and wastelands. It is a perennial that can reach five-feet in height and is topped with pinkish-whitish-purplish flowers.

This antispasmodic, emmenagogue, and sedative has been applied by herbalists for centuries to ameliorate women's disorders. The plant has been used effectively in childbirth and for cases of severe menstrual cramps. It also reputedly eases heart palpitations. However, those sensitive to dermatitis should not handle the plant.

The Japanese believed that the tea made from this plant prolonged life. In the Old English herbals it was attributed with the ability to chase away wicked spirits. In the language of flowers this botanical symbolizes "secret love."

MUGWORT

Names: *Artemisia vulgaris*, **Felon Herb, St. John's Herb. The common name is derived from the fact that the herb was used to flavor beer.**
Associations: Venus, Artemis, Morgana, Neptune.

Mugwort is a type of artemisia. It is a scrubby perennial plant with dusty green leaves and yellow or brown clusters of flowerheads that often grows along roadsides.

In herbal medicine, its properties include emmenagogue, diaphoretic, nervine, diuretic, and stomachic. Acupuncturists prepare moxas of mugwort to cure rheumatism. Sheep like to eat it, and it fattens poultry. Mugwort controls shaking limbs, or what was known in the old days as "quaking of the sinews." It lessens nervous tension arising from PMS, and enables one to sleep. In small doses, this botanical improves the appetite. Like many artemisias, it is used as a moth repellant and is considered poisonous.

This herb provides an essential ingredient in psychic dream pillows. Anoint magic mirrors with distilled mugwort to aid divination. Mugwort and queen-of-the-meadow tea, or simply mugwort steeped in wine, promote clairvoyance and astral projection.

St. John the Baptist was reputed to have worn a girdle of mugwort to protect him from fatigue, sunstroke, wild beasts, evil spirits, and possessions.

In the language of flowers, this botanical symbolizes "happiness." Collect the herb on St. John's Eve, purify it in the bonfire's smoke, and hang it over your doorway to protect the house from evil.

MULLEIN
Names: *Verbascum thapsus,* **Velvet Dock, Bunny's Ears (because the leaves are so soft and downy) Aaron's Rod, Jacob's Staff, Hag's Taper (because formerly it was used to light fires).**
Associations: Jupiter, Saturn.

This ubiquitous botanical of the snapdragon family flourishes in temperate zones along roadsides and in gravelly, sandy areas. By many it is considered a weed. When allowed to grow it becomes a tall hedge plant with pale yellow blossoms and characteristic downy leaves.

As some of the common names for it imply, the ashes help restore gray hair to its original color, and ancient Roman ladies used an infusion of the flowers to bleach their hair. The seeds are said to intoxicate fish when thrown into a river. In this way they enable the fisherman to catch them more easily. The dried stalks can be dipped in candle wax and set ablaze like torches.

The virtues of this botanical include use as an astringent, antispasmodic, demulcent, diuretic, emollient, expectorant, pectoral, vulnerary, sedative, and narcotic. Smoke the dried leaves to help kick the tobacco habit and to soothe mucous membranes irritated from coughing and asthma. The flowers distilled in water alleviate burns, frost bite, piles, and hemorrhoids. Oil of mullein cures earache and destroys germs. A tincture distilled in alcohol suppresses headaches, a decoction of the root is beneficial for gout. It reduces bleeding from lungs and bowels.

Mullein protects against evil spirits and Black Magic. Ulysses is reported to have carried it to insulate himself from the machinations of the Witch, Circe. Burn the leaves in a cauldron in necromancy rituals. It is a prime ingredient of Graveyard Dust.

MUSTARD

Names: *Brassica nigra* (black), *Sinaris alba* (white or yellow).
Associations: Mars, Aries.

A native of the wastelands of Egypt, Syria, and the Mediterranean, the hot, spicy seeds of the white variety are much valued as a condiment. On the other hand, the black seeds are used more often in Magic.

Mustard seed is an alterative, emetic (in large doses), carminative, counterirritant (as a plaster), diuretic, pectoral, rubefacient, stimulant, and antiseptic. It sterilizes and deodorizes, and is good for pains of neuralgia and spasms.

Mustard seeds allegedly keep lovers faithful, protect from danger, and curse enemies when hurled into their doorways.

NETTLE

Names: *Urtica dioica,* Stinging Nettle (so named because the minute hairs that cover the plant sting the skin when merely touched.)
Associations: Mars, Pluto, Aries, Thor (This is why Nordic peasantry sometimes throw nettles on the fire during a thunderstorm in the belief that they will keep from being struck by Thor's lightning bolts.)

Called the scourge of the English countryside, nettle is a persistent and inconvenient weed. The roots render a green dye and when mixed with alum, a yellow dye. The dried, heart-shaped, finely toothed leaves (they lose their sting when dried) are an effective hair tonic, and provide nutritious fodder. The boiled young shoots may be eaten, as the sting also is dissipated by heat. The fiber is spun into a yarn to make fish net and twine. Yellow dock (which often grows near nettle) and plantain are antidotes to the sting.

This valuable, but almost forgotten herb is an alterative, astringent, antiasthmatic, stimulant, expectorant, excellent hemostatic, and tonic. Eat it to help lose weight. Nettle aids the assimilation of minerals; so is doubly good for people on diets. This botanical is rich in iron, therefore, it is beneficial in cases of anemia. The juice stimulates hair growth.

The blame goes to the Romans for first sowing in Britain this plant, now so difficult to eradicate. Legend has it that they did it so they could rub nettles on their bodies to improve their circulation in what they thought was an unbearably cold climate.

In a Hans Christian Anderson tale, a princess weaves eleven coats of nettle for eleven swans. In folklore, it is said that evil spirits will shy away from nettle-fed cattle. Since nettles are prickly the Doctrine of Signatures claims they help relieve uncomfortable situations and stop jealous rumors from spreading.

NUTMEG
Names: *Myristica fragrans,* Nux Moschata.
Associations: Jupiter, Moon, Venus, the Hawaiian pantheon of gods and goddesses.

The kernel of a fruit native to Malaysia, Sumatra, and French Guinea, nutmeg is used as a culinary spice. However, it is poisonous in large doses, and may cause miscarriages.

It is a stimulant to the gastro-intestinal tract, and externally a stimulant for sore muscles and joints. This botanical is also slightly narcotic.

As a key ingredient of love potions, nutmeg was much favored by Napoleon and Josephine. Carry it to increase wealth, improve business, and win the lottery. The hollowed-out kernel filled with mercury and carried in a mojo bag brings good luck.

A unique use for nutmeg given by Sarah Morrison is to place the whole fruit in the corners of a messy room in your house, then chant, "Keep this room from all travail." This allegedly encourages the inhabitant of the room to clean up her/his act.[17] Try it on your teenager and let me know!

Marie Laveau II, a famous Voodoo queen, recommended that ministers wash their church floors with a mixture of ammonia, nutmeg and sugar to attract parishioners.

PARSLEY

Names: *Petroselinum crispum,* **Curly Parsley.**
Associations: Persephone, Mercury.

Parsley is a common kitchen biennial herb of the carrot family, frequently used as a garnish. People used to think that it increased vitality and strength. Perhaps here is one instance of a coincidental relationship between fact and fantasy, as parsley is known to be rich in vitamins A, B-1, B-2, B-3, and C.

Formerly parsley was considered an antidote to poison so that garnishing food with it was symbolic of trust. It is said to make a luxuriant hair rinse.

A laxative, carminative, diuretic, expectorant, and nervine, the herb also is useful in cases of dropsy, jaundice, bites, stings, intestinal gas, bladder infections, kidney stones, and scrofulous swellings. Parsley is said to help dispel tumors and sweeten the breath.

This plant is reputed to have sprung from the blood of the Greek hero, Arcturus, who as a child, was swallowed by a snake while resting on a parsley leaf. An offertory herb in ancient Greek funeral rites, parsley often was placed on tombs of the dead to bring them good luck in the Afterworld. Parsley is also a typical ingredient in the "pay off" meals that Voodoo practitioners leave for the gods to thank them for requests granted.

The crispy leaves were fashioned into victors' crowns at ancient Greek games, as they were considered the symbol of strength. Parsley is believed to urge on race horses, and is an ingredient of love philtres to bewitch the opposite sex.

PASSION FLOWER

Names: *Passiflora incarnata,* **Passion Vine, Apricot Vine, Maypop.**
Associations: Sun, Neptune.

Named for the Passion of Christ, Christians see in the features of the purple flowers of this climbing vine the symbols of the Crucifixion. The corona in the center particularly resembles the crown of thorns. Some species bear a yellow fruit from which a delicious juice is extracted.

This antispasmodic, nervine, and sedative, is a narcotic painkiller in cases of dysmenorrhea. Passion flower restores frazzled nerves and counteracts insomnia and hysteria.

The flower brings good luck in love. If you carry the dried flower, it is alleged to prevent others' anger from affecting you. In the language of flowers, this plant refers to "belief."

PATCHOULY
Names: *Pogostemon patchouli,* **also spelled Patchouli.**
Associations: Exu (Brazil), Scorpio, Pluto.

An insect repellant of the mint family, this herbaceous shrub native to India has a distinctively earthy smell considered by some a pleasant inhalant, and by others an obnoxious odor. It was used to keep away insects and moths from Indian shawls in the nineteenth century.

Paradoxically, patchouly is believed to possess the power both to win love and drive away enemies, but also to separate lovers. It is an essential component of Graveyard Dust, and many Black Magic and uncrossing spells.

PENNYROYAL
Name: *Mentha pulegium.*
Associations: Jupiter, Venus.

The oil of this pungent mint is an insect repellant that soothes itchy skin. I do not recommend it for internal use by pregnant women because it is a strong abortive.

Pennyroyal protects against the evil eye and seasickness, and helps keep the spark of love kindled between husband and wife.

PEONY
Names: *Paeonia genus.* **This plant is named for the Greek physician, Paeon, who cured Pluto of wounds he received in the Trojan war. It is also an epithet for Apollo because he applied the plant to cure the gods' wounds.**
Associations: Moon, Pluto, Venus.

Because the peony is an easily grown, low bush with large, fragrant pink, white, or red flowers, it often is used in home landscaping. Unfortunately, the blooms are short-lived, and don't dry well for fragrance-crafting.

An antispasmodic, nervine, and tonic, it is recommended for headache, epileptic convulsions, and liver obstructions.

Peony flowers bring good luck. The seeds are a charm against evil spirits and nightmares. To make a wish come true, write your request on parchment with red ink, and sprinkle it with dried pink peony flowers. Roll up the parchment, tie it with red yarn, and hide it in a drawer until your desire is fulfilled. Afterwards, burn the entire parchment.

PEPPERMINT

Name: *Mentha piperita.*
Associations: Jupiter, Venus, Persephone, Pluto.
One of the many kinds of hardy perennial mints that grow throughout the temperate zones, peppermint is an edible garnish, seasoning, and ingredient in candy, lozenges, and herbal beverage teas.

Peppermint is known as an antispasmodic, disinfectant, and nervine. It relieves symptoms of colds, flu, insomnia, toothache, headache, rheumatism, and sore throat. Rats avoid it because they dislike the odor.

The Greeks and Romans crowned their leaders and heroes with peppermint wreaths. Allegedly, the herb protects against evil Witches and vampires. Use a drop of the oil to activate any spell. When drunk as a tea before bedtime, the herb encourages prophetic dreams. Peppermint (along with ash, basil, periwinkle, sage and vervain) was used by ancient Celts to purify water for rituals.

PERIWINKLE

Names: *Vinca minor,* **Sorcerer's Violet, Ground Ivy. It is sometimes called Myrtle, and therefore is confused with the Myrtle Tree, or California Laurel (***Umbellularia Californica***).**
Association: Moon.
This perennial evergreen plant of the dogbane family has glossy, dark green, oval-shaped leaves with blue, violet, or white five-petaled flowers. It grows best in the shade as a ground cover.

The botanical is considered poisonous by the FDA, so I do not recommend you prescribe it medicinally. Traditionally, it was applied as a hemostatic, laxative, astringent, and tonic. As an ointment it works well for piles and skin inflammations. Carefully administered, it staunches bleeding and cramps, and is beneficial for diabetes and high blood pressure.

Periwinkle is an ingredient of love charms and philtres. The French associate it with pleasant memories and friendship. The herb is used in spells to recall past lives, especially when mixed with Mystic Rites incense. However, it also is considered a flower of death, as periwinkle garlands formerly wreathed children's coffins.

PLANTAIN

Names: *Plantago major, P. lanceolata,* Englishman's-foot. The Irish call this plant *Slan-lus,* which means "healing herb."
Associations: Venus, Saturn, Mars.

Plantain flourishes at the roadsides and in wastelands. It grows on long stalks one- to two-feet high, and shows broad, oval leaves and spikes of yellowish-white or greenish-brown flowers. Do not confuse this plant with the similarly named *platano* (plane tree), as they are two very different botanicals.

It is an astringent (the leaves contain tannin), anti- inflammatory, diuretic (*P. major),* and hemostatic. Use it to heal cuts, sores, boils, and snake and insect bites. The seeds can be brewed in a tea to cure dysentery and bleeding from mucous membranes.

Plantain is one of the plants called the mother of herbs, and is highly respected by Witch healers. In the Anglo-Saxon Charm of the Nine Herbs, plantain is said to deflect "the venom that flies through the air, and the loathed things that through the land rove."

POPPY

Names: *Papaver rhoeas,* Corn Poppy, Red Poppy; *Eschscholzia californica,* California Poppy; *Papaver somniferum* Opium Poppy, White Poppy; *Argemone mexicana,* Mexican Poppy, Yellow Prickly Poppy. These flowers all belong to the same poppy family.
Associations: Moon (white), Saturn (black), Capricorn (black), Aries (red), Sun (yellow).

Opium is extracted from the unripe heads of the strongly narcotic white poppy. The red poppy contains some of the same properties as the white, but in much lesser concentration. Other than its well-known hypnotic, narcotic, and sedative properties, the poppy is a reputed analgesic, astringent, antispasmodic, diaphoretic, and expectorant. Poppy heads of the white variety contain morphine, narcotine, and codeine.

Poppies are an emblem of those who have died in war. This is why they are worn on Veteran's Day. Place red poppy seeds on hot coals and inhale the incense to glimpse the future. The seeds are alleged to cause quarrels.

QUEEN-OF-THE-MEADOW
Names: *Filipendula ulmaria,* **Meadowsweet, Bridewort.**
Associations: Gemini, Jupiter, the Druids.

This well-known botanical of the rose family with creamy white flower clusters and fern-like foliage similar to that of a wildflower can grow quite tall. The leaves are almond-scented, and in former times were strewn on the floor to perfume the house, especially bedrooms. Meadowsweet comprises an ingredient of mead (the name is a corruption of the term "meadsweet"), and herb beers.

An astringent, diuretic, and tonic, it checks diarrhea and dropsy, and is considered an effective diet tea. The plant contains salicylic acid, a key ingredient of aspirin.

This sacred herb of the Druids supposedly brings visions of the future when brewed and drunk as a tea, or when added to the bath. Lay queen-of-the-meadow around the circumference of the Circle to invite the blessings of the Lord and Lady. Add a pint of water distilled with one tablespoon of this botanical to your bath before going out in search of a job.

RASPBERRY
Name: *Rubus idaeus.*
Associations: Jupiter, Venus.

This prickly bush that grows near water is famous for its sweet, red or black berries. The berries can be transformed into wine, preserves, brandy, vinegar, beverage teas, and red dye — that is, if you succeed in collecting enough berries and don't pop them all in your mouth!

The leaves are an antispasmodic, astringent, and stimulant known as one of the best herbal teas to relieve the cramps of menses.

Raspberry leaves attenuate nausea in pregnancy, prevent hemorrhage, and ease childbirth. The leaves are good for stomach complaints, fevers, colds, flus, and canker sores. Make it into a poultice along with slippery elm to cleanse wounds.

In the language of flowers this botanical represents "remorse."

ROSE

Name: *Rosa genus.*
Associations: Venus, Jupiter, Adonis, Libra (white), Moon (wild rose).

The rose is probably the most universally recognized and beloved flower. Rosehips (the mature seed head) contain large amounts of vitamin C. The flower petals make an unusual edible garnish. Roses are valued for their scent in perfumes, potpourris, incenses, sachets, scented beads, and cosmetics, including skin care products. If you want to read more about the different kinds of roses and their applications in fragrance-crafting, read my book, *Witch's Brew.*

The petals are an astringent, emmenagogue, stomachic, and mild laxative, and are useful in cough syrup. Rosewater cures watery eye inflammations and lung hemorrhages. Employ roses to increase semen and cure vomiting.

The rose is an emblem of high aspiration in several religions and magical sects including Christianity, Rosicrucianism, Qabalism, and Freemasonry. Rose buds symbolize love and devotion. For good luck, throw the buds on an open fire.

To meet a new love, make a sachet of powdered rosebuds, mint, and musk crystals. Add twenty-one drops of rose oil, and seven drops of musk oil, and one drop of peppermint oil, and rub on your hands before going out. To revitalize your love life, sprinkle rosewater on the bed.

ROSEMARY

Names: *Rosmarinus officinalis,* **Incensier, Old Man.**
Associations: Virgin Mary, St. Magdalene, Sun.

This shrubby, tender perennial of the mint family displays needle-like leaves that emit a pungent scent, somewhat like camphor. Rosemary water makes a superior hair rinse that removes soapy residue and prevents hair from falling out. It is also a spicy condiment and fumigant. Fragrant rosemary wreaths used to decorate staircases at Christmastime.

This botanical is an antispasmodic, astringent, diaphoretic, carminative, and stomachic. It purifies the sick room, and is considered a restorative in nervous diseases, colds, and fevers. It alleviates flatulence, asthma, colic, nausea, kidney disorders and headaches. The herb is a nutritive, rich in easily assimilable calcium. Rosemary also cleanses the intestines.

Burn rosemary with thyme in Druidic rites. As a link to bind together members of your Coven, give each member of the group a sprig of fresh rosemary tied with a colorful ribbon at the Winter Solstice. It is an effective uncrossing herb that drives away evil, purifies the atmosphere, soothes the troubled spirit and attracts positive influences.

It symbolizes fidelity to lovers, for as the age-old saying goes, "Rosemary is for remembrance." It was formerly also the custom in Wales for people to remember the dead by carrying garlands of rosemary to funerals and placing them on graves before lowering them into the ground.

Rosemary adds power to any spell. Along with thyme and verbena, it is a principal ingredient of Holy Water. This botanical is alleged to strengthen the memory. Rub a thief's feet with the oil to take away his will to steal.

RUE

Names: *Ruta graveolens*, Herb of Grace (this name originated with the use of rue brushes by the Roman Catholic Church to sprinkle Holy Water), Countryman's-treacle.
Associations: Sun, Diana in *la vecchia religione* of Italy.

A hardy evergreen, the yellow flowers form groups of four, crowned by one group of five at the top of each branch, which leads to the association of the plant with the symbol of the pentagram.

Rue is an abortifacient, antispasmodic, emmenagogue, rubefacient, stimulant, and tonic for mental stress. It dispels fatigue, soothes tired eyes, and cures weakness in muscles. This botanical also guards against dizziness, congestion, rheumatism, heart palpitations, piles, kidney disorders, cramps, and hypertension. Apply it as a compress to the chest to calm bronchial coughs. However, do not ingest it if you are pregnant.

One of the bitter herbs of the Hebrews, rue is a symbol of grief and regret. The botanical is an important protection herb in Witchcraft. It is alleged to improve clairvoyance. If ingested in a tea, rue is instrumental in spells to hold a lover or to strengthen the will. It is an ingredient of Voodoo Four Thieves Vinegar.

SAFFRON

Names: *Crocus sativus.*
Associations: Sun, Leo.

Saffron is a yellow substance found in the pistils of the flower of a kind of crocus. It is a very expensive commodity, as it takes 60,000 stigmas to make one pound of saffron. The pistils yield a yellow dye, and are prized as a culinary spice. It is a diaphoretic, emmenagogue, and hemostatic, especially effective in stemming uterine hemorrhages.

The Greek gods and goddesses always dressed in saffron-hued robes. By analogy, saffron may be added in petitions to the gods. The Romans valued a blend of saffron and other herbs as a cordial and as a cardiac and sexual stimulant. Zeus and Hera's marriage bed was said to be made of saffron. Sprinkle it on Voodoo dolls to make a person do your bidding. Safflower (*Carthamus tinctorius*) or marigold flowers may be substituted for saffron in rituals.

SAGE

Names: *Salvia officinalis*. The Latin genus name means "healthy."
Associations: Jupiter, Venus, Leo.

Sage is an evergreen of the mint family native to the Mediterranean with grayish-green leaves and blue-violet flowers. Of the many types, the wild variety native to Colorado imparts a particularly fresh scent to our high meadows, and by extension, to woodsy potpourris and sachets. It is a condiment and flavoring for wine and ale.

The leaves are an antispasmodic, antipyretic, astringent, carminative, and stimulant. An infusion of the leaves will slow the flow of bodily excretions such as night sweats, postnasal drip, and blood. Formerly this herb was used to dress open wounds. It eliminates canker sores and nervous headaches, soothes itchy skin, and purifies the liver and kidneys. Prevent a cold by boiling sage with lemon and honey and imbibe the brew as a beverage tea. It is said to ease the soreness of tonsillitis.

Sage allegedly confers wisdom (hence, the name) when drunk daily as a tea. Hang it from your front door and replace monthly to absorb negativity. It is an ancient symbol of immortality that was employed in rituals to drives away evil. The herb is said to thrive or wither in the garden according the fortunes of the one who tends it. Another piece of folklore states that where sage thrives in the garden, the wife rules the roost!

SAINT JOHN'S-WORT
Names: *Hypericum perforatum*, Aaron's Beard, Amber Touch-and-heal, Rosin Rose, Goatweed, Klamath Weed. This favorite botanical of medieval monastery gardens is named for the apostle, John, because it flowers around St. John's Day.
Association: Sun.

It is a woody-stemmed plant that grows in pastures and meadows; the flowers have yellow petals with black dots at the margins.

The plant is considered poisonous by the FDA, but traditionally, herbalists prescribe it as an astringent, diuretic, expectorant, vulnerary, and nervine. The herb is alleged to relieve nervous exhaustion and prevent bed-wetting. It has been applied in cases of catarrh, diarrhea, pulmonary congestion, jaundice, subcutaneous bleeding, and paralysis due to stroke.

Jump over a flowering St. John's-wort plant at midnight on the Summer Solstice to become fertile. Place the dried leaves inside a mojo bag and hang it around your neck as a an amulet. Try adding it to love potions, or use a distillation of this botanical in your floorwash to keep peace in the home.

The Greeks believed that a whiff of the herb would cause evil spirits to vanish and would protect them from thunder. In ancient times, St. John's-wort was thought to cure insanity and melancholy.

SAVORY
Names: *Satureja hortensis* (Summer Savory is an annual),
***S. montana* (Winter Savory is a perennial).**
Associations: Mercury, Sun.

The leaves of this foot-tall, woody herb with tiny white, pink, or lilac flowers are used to flavor bean and pea dishes. The plant is one of the many members of the mint family, and is related to sage and thyme. Once it was classified as a kind of thyme.

Savory is a carminative rich in potassium, and is used by herbalists to cure women's complaints. A cupful of tea brewed from the fresh leaves and consumed each day is supposed to be slimming.

Summer savory was known formerly as the "sex herb," while the winter variety was considered a sexual depressant. In Italy, mothers would feed the summer variety to their daughters for a month before the wedding so they would please their husbands. A sprig tucked into the bridal bouquet is alleged to insure fertility. In former times in French hotels, the hoteliers would place a dish of summer savory and a bottle of champagne beside the nuptial bed. On the other hand, wives used to put winter savory in their husbands' salads so they would fall asleep quickly after dinner.

SKULLCAP
Names: *Scutellaria lateriflora*, Blue Pimpernel, Mad-dog Weed, Scullcap, Helmetflower. This botanical receives its generic name from a Latin word meaning "little duck," because of the calyx which forms a bulging upper lid on the lower lip like a lid on a hinge. The flower also looks like a type of military helmet with the visor raised.
Associations: Virgo, Saturn.

The twelve- to eighteen-inch tall creeping perennial with oblong opposite downy leaves is considered an antipyretic, antispasmodic, astringent, nervine, and tonic. This herb of the mint family helps cure hysteria, convulsions, St. Vitus's dance, rickets, neuralgia, headaches caused by coughing, and nervous headaches. It alleviates alcohol withdrawal symptoms and counteracts sterility. It is prized as a nutritive high in calcium, magnesium, and potassium.

If worn in a sachet by a woman, or introduced into her husband's food, skullcap will keep him true. Use it in a spell when you need to obtain a loan.

SENNA
Names: *Cassia senna; Cassia marilandica*, American Senna, Locust Plant, Maryland Cassia, Wild Senna.
Association: Saturn.

This member of the pea family forms elongated seedpods that when dried make an interesting addition to potpourris. Senna grows

in thickets, at roadsides, and in dry areas. It is a four-foot tall perennial with pinnately compound leaves in four to eight pairs, and
bright yellow flowers with brown centers.

It is a cathartic (in large doses) and laxative (the leaves). The root
can be pounded into a poultice to relieve sores.

According to Aima in *Ritual Book of Herbal Spells,*[18] an incense
made from powdered senna and John the conqueror root will influence people in your favor. Carry the leaves to make people more
favorably disposed to you. Anoint your lover's thighs with the tea to
keep love true.

SNAKEROOT

**Names: *Aristolochia serpentaria,* Birthwort, Pelican Flower,
Sangreal, Snakeweed, Virginia Snakeroot, Texas Snakeroot.
Associations: The North American Indian gods, the pantheon of the
Southern United States Voodun deities.**

Snakeroot grows in the Central and Southern United States. It
receives its name from its large, twisting root structure. The plant
exhibits a long, tubular, brownish-purple flower and heart-shaped
leaves that exude a fetid odor.

It is a diaphoretic, stimulant, and tonic. Small doses encourage
the appetite and tone the digestive organs, but large doses cause
nausea and cramps in the bowels, and genetic mutations in fetuses.
This botanical is beneficial in cases of typhoid fever, dyspepsia, and
amenorrhea.

Snakeroot is effective in spells to rid yourself of an enemy or
unwanted suitor. It is also an ingredient of money spells.

SOLOMON'S SEAL

**Names: *Polygonatum biflorum, P. multiflorum, P. officinale* (Euro-
pean species), St. Mary's Seal. Its name originated in the belief that
wise King Solomon himself revealed this herb to the benefit of
humanity.
Association: Saturn.**

As a member of the lily family, Solomon's seal is often confused
with this more common, poisonous garden plant, but can be distinguished by its greater height, white flowers that hang in pairs, and
black berries. The fleshy root is the part used.

It is an antiemetic, hemostatic, and restorative tonic, excellent for female complaints. It assuages inflammation of the stomach and bowels, is good for pulmonary consumption, checks dysentery, and helps cure skin abrasions.

Solomon's seal is a beneficial herb in exorcism and house-blessing rituals. The flowers are a love potion ingredient.

SOUTHERNWOOD
Names: *Artemisia abrotanum,* **Lad's Love (this name derives from the fact that in times gone by, boys made an ointment of southernwood and spread it on their faces in hopes of growing beards).**
Associations: Mercury, Aquarius.

The leaves of this artemisia, similar in appearance to mugwort, can be either camphor-, lemon- or thyme-scented, which makes it a valuable addition to potpourris.

The leaves are an emmenagogue, nervine, stimulant, and tonic. When boiled in barley meal and used in an emollient on the face, the mixture helps eradicate pimples. The plant also eliminates worms in children and relieves eye inflammations. Remember, as an artemisia, southernwood is somewhat poisonous.

Southernwood is a traditional ingredient of love and fidelity spells. Stuff it in your matress to make your lover's passion everlasting. In the language of flowers, this botanical stands for "jest" and "bantering."

SPIKENARD
Names: *Aralia racemosa,* **American Sarsparilla, Indian Root,**
Association: Aquarius.

It is a tall plant of the ginseng family that can grow up to ten feet high. It renders a fragrant, spicy oil through its roots which is difficult to obtain from botanical supplies houses.

Wild spikenard, *A. nudicaulis,* is an alterative (particularly for syphilis), diaphoretic, and stimulant. It increases energy levels so the body can fight pulmonary infections and rheumatism.

Make a decoction of the root and anoint the picture of your loved one with the liquid to insure lifelong fidelity.

STRAWBERRY

Name: *Fragaria genus.*
Associations: Libra, Venus.

Everyone knows the gastronomic delights of fat, juicy strawberries, but the plant was also a popular cosmetics ingredient long before the advent of the Body Shop. Strawberry is used both as a fragrance and as a facial to tighten pores. To remove yellow stains from your teeth, apply strawberry and raspberry juice to them, wait five minutes, and clean off with bicarbonate of soda and warm water.

This botanical of the rose family is an anti-abortive, astringent, diuretic, and laxative. The juice relieves sunburn pain, the leaves in a beverage tea make a fine female tonic, and of course, the berry are a favorite jam and jelly.

Gather the leaves on Lammas Eve and distill them into an exotic perfume to entice gnomes to the Magic Circle. They just can't seem to resist! In the language of flowers, this botanical signifies "perfect excellence."

TANSY

Names: *Tanacetum vulgare,* **Buttons, Goose Tansy. The name is a corruption of a Greek word meaning "immortality."**
Associations: Jupiter, Gemini, Venus.

Tansy is a bitter, aromatic plant with clusters of close, small-headed yellow flowers that look like buttons; hence the name "buttons."

It is considered both an abortive and a poison by the FDA, so internal use is not recommended. Its properties include use as an emmenagogue, tonic, stimulant, febrifuge, diaphoretic, and nervine. It is alleged to dispel intestinal worms and to be beneficial in cases of hysteria, kidney weakness, and eruptive skin disorders. For gout, prepare an infusion, and soak your foot in it. Tansy is an excellent moth repellant and air freshener. This is one of the bitter herbs the Hebrews eat in small amounts at Passover.

TARRAGON

Names: Artemisia dracunculus, Dragon's-mugwort, Dragon Herb, French Tarragon, Little Dragon.
Association: Mars.

Tarragon is a five-foot tall, perennial of the artemisia family identified by its woody stem and coiling root, narrow leaves with an anise-like odor, and tiny yellow flowers that bear no seeds. It is a culinary herb used to flavor meat, fish, chicken, salads, dressings, and sauce bernaise. A Russian variety exists that looks similar, but has little taste and does bear seeds.

Tarragon is an emmenagogue, diuretic, aperient, and ancient antidote for the bites of venomous animals. It is supposed to soothe rheumatism and arthritis. The oil is alleged to cure certain cancers if taken in large doses over long periods of time. The Egyptians applied the juice from the crushed leaves externally to clear dark circles from under their eyes.

Tarragon is known as dragon herb because it allegedly sprung from the path the serpent took on leaving the Garden of Eden. Arab kings thought it improved their love-making performance. Marie Antoinette each day commanded her gardener to find the most perfect leaves for her salad to be picked with white kid gloves at dawn; hence the expression "to handle with kid gloves."

THYME

Names: *Thymus vulgaris* (Garden Thyme), *T. serpyllum* (Wild Thyme, also called Mother of Thyme, Creeping Thyme), *T. citriodorus* (Lemon Thyme). The name is derived from a Greek term meaning "to fumigate."
Associations: Venus, Sun, Saturn.

The Romans used this hardy, creeping, fragrant herb to flavor cheeses and liqueurs. Its balsamic odor makes it an ideal addition to incense, potpourris, and sachets. Plant mini-thyme between the stones of the walkway to your flower or herb garden to prevent weeds.

The leaves are an antiseptic, antispasmodic, antitussive, carminative, diaphoretic, expectorant, and tonic. It is a parasiticide for intestinal worms, lice, crabs, and skin parasites, and destroys fungal infections like athletes' foot.

The ancient Greeks saw in thyme a symbol of bravery, courage, energy, and graceful elegance. Add it to money spells and charm bags to bring fast luck. It is an ingredient of house blessing rites. Carry thyme so others will praise your actions. Wild thyme invokes the fairies. Women wear this botanical in a sachet between the breasts to keep their husbands faithful.

It is yet another reputed aphrodisiac, and in ancient times was given to young girls who had just begun menses so that they would soon become interested in men, lose their virginity, and perhaps be saved from being sacrificed to propitiate the gods.

TONKA BEAN
Names: *Dipteryx odorata,* Tonquin Bean.
Associations: Erzulie (Haiti), Iemanjá (Brazil), Gemini.

The seed of this Brazilian tree, called a bean, exudes a fragrant odor of vanilla and almonds that lends a lovely scent to potpourris, sachets, and incenses. It is also a fixative for these blends.

The beans are highly poisonous and will paralyze the heart, so I do not recommend their application in herbal medicine. However, traditionally, they were used as a cardiac and narcotic.

Carry a bean to attract love and protect you from illness, or add it to a prosperity charm. In Voodoo, tonka beans are called "wish beans," and if tossed in the water, are believed to make dreams come true.

UVA-URSI
Names: *Arctostaphylos uva-ursi, Arbutus uva-ursi,* Kinnikinnick, Bearberry, Bear's-grape, Crowberry, Foxberry, Hog Cranberry, Mealberry, Upland Cranberry. The various names associated with this plant show its popularity with wildlife.
Association: Libra.

The dried, dark green, leathery leaves of this trailing evergreen of the heath family are the part used. The leaves yield an ash-colored dye, and are a tanning agent in Russian leather.

They also are alterative, astringent, and diuretic, and helpful for disorders of the bladder and kidney. They can be prescribed as a postpartum tonic for the womb. Uva-ursi is also said to cure cystitis and venereal diseases.

Uva-ursi invokes the Dryads (spirits that dwell in trees) and aids divination. It is also used in incense-making with wood betony, frankincense, sandalwood, nutmeg, and orris powder to help improve the mental faculties. Leave it in an open dish on the altar to aid astral projection and general magical work.

VALERIAN

Names: *Valeriana officinalis,* All-heal, Garden Heliotrope, Setwell, Vandalroot.
Associations: Venus, Virgo, Mercury.

Valerian is found in damp spots in woods, hedges, river banks, and at the roadside in the Northern temperate zone. The peculiar, fetid odor of the root is irresistible to cats and rats. In fact, it probably was the herb the Pied Piper of Hamelin used to rid his town of rats. On the other hand, the pink or white flowers, standing in clusters atop long stems and flanked by feathery leaves have a heavenly scent.

The root is a nervine, sedative, carminative, antispasmodic, and stimulant. It is excellent for nervous complaints, insomnia, and headaches. It relieves cramps, pains, stomach gas, epilepsy, and convulsions. Valerian root slows and strengthens the heartbeat.

It is a component of Graveyard Dust and an ingredient in charms to restore peace and harmony to the home. Inhale the crushed root in an incense, or drink the tea to produce prophetic dreams.

VERBENA

Names: *Aloysia triphylla,* Lemon Verbena, Herb Louisa, Van Van (a Voodoo anointing oil).
Association: Venus.

It is a shrub with lemon-scented leaves native to Chile. An antispasmodic, carminative, stomachic, and sedative. It treats dyspepsia, indigestion, and flatulence. Use it in a wash to clear acne.

An ingredient of love charms and Holy Water, lemon verbena is said to drive away evil influences and attract positive vibrations if carried in charm bag. However, do not hang verbena in your door-way or it will cause family relationships to disintegrate.

Add it to your bath water before going to an interview— espe-cially an audition in the arts—as it will increase your poise and self-assurance. Mix one tablespoon each of verbena leaves, linden flowers, saffron, cinnamon, nutmeg, powdered rose petals, and one-half teaspoon of saltpeter, and burn in an incense to start your creative juices flowing so you can better perform music, write, dance, paint, or act.

VERVAIN

Names: *Verbena officinalis,* **Simplers Joy, Fit Plant, Herb-of-the-cross (it was said to have staunched Christ's wounds), Pigeon's-grass, Mercury's Blood, Tears of Isis, Enchanter's Plant.**
Associations: Venus, Diana, Demeter, Persephone, Juno, Gemini, the Druids.

It is a spiky plant with coarse-toothed or lanced and opposite leaves, and five-petaled red, purplish, or white flowers.

Vervain possesses the qualities of an antispasmodic, antipyretic, astringent, diaphoretic, expectorant, nervine, vermicide, and diuretic, and contains vitamin K. This botanical helps ease wheezy breathing and cures headaches, gout, jaundice, and gallstones. Use it as an eyewash and throat gargle. It successfully eliminates blood in the urine.

A love herb, it is potent in any kind of love and fertility Magic. This is why in the old days German brides wore it in their hair. Also include it in spells to overcome fear. Ambassadors carried sprigs of vervain when negotiating with enemies, as it was alleged to overcome any enmity.

The Romans burned this herb to purify their temples and houses. Steep it in wash water, and clean your house with it to protect the inhabitants from harm. Supposedly it possesses the virtue of granting wishes in all categories, and especially attracts new love. Vervain invokes the protective force of the Moon goddess and helps make one fertile in body and mind. In the language of flowers, the plant aptly means "enchantment."

VIOLET

Names: *Viola odorata,* **Sweet Violet, Blue Violet, English Violet.**
Associations: Libra, Aphrodite.

The tiny, extremely fragrant, purple or white flowers bloom in April. Violets spread easily through the grass and garden. Some butterflies feed exclusively on their sweet nectar. The flowers are prized in perfumery, and can be crystallized into a sweet violet sugar. The raw flowers also make a pretty, edible garnish.

An expectorant, diuretic, and slight laxative, it also flavors and neutralizes the acidic taste of medicines. The rhizome is a strong purgative alleged to cure skin cancer and cancer of the tongue.

When Jupiter, out of fear of Juno's jealousy, changed Io into a white heifer, the violet flower sprang from the field, and became her food. It is an ingredient in love and enchantment spells. Put a thin layer of violet flowers in your shoes to attract a lover or to reunite yourself with a lost love. Place them in a bowl by a sick person's bed to draw healing vibration. The ancient Greeks thought that the calming effects of the scent of violets moderated anger. The Greeks also associated the flower with the death of the young and premature death. Conversely, it is believed that to keep a violet plant in the house attracts good luck.

WOODRUFF
Names: *Asperula odorata,* **Sweet Woodruff, Master-of-the-wood, Waldmeister.**
Associations: Mars, the Fairies.

Woodruff is a short, hardy perennial herb about a foot high with small white flowers that bloom in May. It likes the shade of the woods, hence its name. People stuffed mattresses and pillows with the herb because of its hay-like scent. The botanical still is used to scent linens and to fix the scent of some perfumes. Woodruff was often employed during the Middle Ages as an herbal remedy. It is an antiarthritic and laxative.

Place a sprig of fresh woodruff in the Maibowle on Beltane along with a fruity white wine, sugar, carbonated water, strawberries, and pieces of pineapple. Drink and rejoice! Strew the fragrant leaves about the house to freshen the rooms and protect yourself from psychic attack. Put the leaves in your closet to draw the blessings of the wee folk.

YARROW
Names: *Achillea millefolium,* **Bloodwort, Knight's Milfoil (this name, meaning a "thousand leaves" refers to its feathery leaves), Sanguinary, Stanchgrass.**
Associations: Venus, Gemini.

The herb, with its closely formed yellow or white flowerheads and feathery leaves on sturdy stalks, abounds in meadows and sunny mountain slopes.

The flowers are an anti-inflammatory, astringent, antipyretic, diaphoretic, antibacterial, carminative, hemostatic, mild stimulant, and vulnerary. The Highlanders of Scotland and ancient Greeks used to make an ointment from the plant to cure wounds. Chew the leaves to alleviate toothaches. Yarrow tea remedies severe colds. It is a blood purifier that also staunches nosebleeds.

Formerly this herb was thought to belong to the Devil.

Drink the tea to dispel melancholy. Place yarrow under your pillow so that a vision of your true love will appear to you in a dream. Yarrow sticks instead of coins may be employed in the I Ching method of divination, and in my experience, seem more accurate.

YELLOW DOCK

Names: *Rumex crispus,* **Curled Dock.**
Association: Aries.

A yellow-rooted plant that often grows near nettles, it is a cure for their sting. The plant is treated as a tenacious garden weed. Yellow dock is also an alterative, mild tonic, astringent, nutritive, cholagogue, and laxative. It is useful in cases of jaundice, piles, rheumatism, chronic skin diseases, and bleeding from the lungs.

Wash the doorknobs of your store with yellow dock tea to attract business. The herbal healers of Anglo-Saxon England used to mix yellow dock with Holy Water and ale to cure people of the infamous disease they called "elf-shot."

YERBA SANTA

Names: *Eriodictyon californicum,* **Holy Herb, Mountain Balm.**
Association: the Great Mother.

It is a low, shrubby evergreen, native to the dry hills of northern Mexico and southern California. This botanical is known as an astringent, expectorant, stimulant, and bitter tonic. It is good for bronchitis, laryngitis, and pulmonary infections.

Carry it to increase your spiritual strength and to receive the blessings of the goddess. This botanical grants you the power to defeat the forces of evil.

Appendices

I. Medical Terms

abortifacient - A substance that induces a miscarriage.

alterative - A blood purifier that treats toxicity in blood. An alterative "alters" the condition of a disease. It also cure infections, arthritis, cancer, skin eruptions, etc.

amenorrhea - A condition of absence of menstruation; i.e., where a woman is unable to have a period.

analgesic - Something that temporarily relieves pain without producing loss of consciousness. Some analgesics work generally on the brain or nerves, while others have a local effect.

anodyne - A substance that relieves pain and usually also induces sleep.

antacid - A remedy that neutralizes excess acid in the stomach and intestines.

anthelmintic - A substance that destroys intestinal worms.

antiabortive - An agent that prevents pregnant woman from miscarrying.

anti-asthmatic - A medicine that allays the paroxysms of asthma attacks.

antibiotic - A substance that literally "kills life" by inhibiting the growth of, or destroying harmful bacteria, viruses, and amoebas. It stimulates the body's own immune response. Helpful bacteria are not affected.

anticatarrhal - An agent that eliminates or counteracts irritated mucous membranes and accompanying sore throat, hoarseness, and coughing.

anti-inflammatory - An agent that reduces the swelling, heat, and pain associated with inflammations.

antipyretic - A fever preventative, or a substance that decreases fevers. Antipyretics neutralize acids and reduce the patient's temperature.

antiseptic - An agent applied to skin to destroy or prevent bacterial growth, sepsis, and putrefication. If the substance is herbal, it will prevent new growth only.

antispasmodic - A substance that prevents or diminishes muscle spasms, cramps, convulsions, and nervous tension. Apply internally or externally for relief.

antitussive - A cough inhibitor.

aphrodisiac - A tonic that improves sexual potency and power.

aromatic - A substance with a fragrant, spicy smell used to make other drugs more palatable.

astringent - Something that constricts and binds soft tissues. It is used to check internal and external secretions like diarrhea and bleeding.

blood purifier - A term used in herbal medicine that applies to a detoxifying agent that neutralizes the acidity in the blood that builds up from the presence of toxic substances which have not been adequately eliminated in the small intestine.

cardiac - A heart tonic; having to do with the heart.

carminative - A medicine that relieves pains in the bowels and expels gas. The word in Latin, carmen, means a "charm."

catarrh - An inflammation of the nasal mucous membranes.

cathartic - A strong laxative.

cholagogue - A substance that increases the flow and discharge of bile from the gall bladder into the small intestine. A "biliar" is a tonic that stimulates the flow of bile. Bile is a liquid stored in the gall bladder that helps digest fat.

decoction - A strong tea that is boiled slowly for at least fifteen to twenty minutes, then strained to render an extract. It is usually made from roots, barks, and/or large seeds of plants.

demulcent - A soothing mucilage that protects internally damaged or inflamed tissues or mucous membranes, quells coughs, lubricates joints, bones, counteracts pain, and encourages healing of the alimentary canal.

diaphoretic - An agent to induce or increase perspiration. It is used against fevers and inflammations, particularly when the skin feels hard and dry.

diuretic - A urinary tonic that increases flow of urine (when taken as a cold tea), and a demulcent to buffer the effect on the kidneys.

douche - A liquid flushed into the vagina, usually for cleansing purposes.

dropsy - A term once used to describe edema, i.e., systemic water retention.

electuary - Also called a "confection," it is an herb or drug mixed with honey, sugar, peanut butter, or syrup, to make it more palatable.

elixir - A sweetened liquid medicine that contains alcohol.

emetic - A medicine to promote vomiting. Use emetics when poisons or excess mucus have accumulated in the body. Avoid them when the patient is extremely ill, as emetics reduce the body's energy level.

emmenagogue - A substance to induce and increase menstrual flow.

emollient - A skin dressing or ointment that soothes, softens, and protects the skin. For example, emollients are useful for relief of eczema.

expectorant - A medicine that expels mucus from the respiratory tract by promoting coughing.

extract - A plant preparation, usually of semi-solid consistency, sometimes containing many plant substances. To prepare an extract, put four ounces of dried or eight ounces of fresh, bruised herbs into a bottle and mix with one part vinegar, alcohol, or massage oil. Shake twice a day for three to fourteen days. Add vitamin E as a preservative, or a grain alcohol, like vodka or gin.

febrifuge - A remedy to allay fevers.

fomentation - Any hot compress applied to the surface of the body with a cloth. It may be moist or dry. Fomentations dilate blood vessels, relieve pain, soften skin, draw out abscesses, and quiet the nerves.

fungicide - A remedy that destroys fungus.

galactogogue - A substance that increases secretion of milk in nursing mothers.

hemostatic - An agent that arrests internal or external hemorrhaging.

hepatic - A tonic for the liver.

homeopathy - A system of medicine based on the aspect of the theory of the Doctrine of Signatures where it is believed that "like cures like." Minute doses of medicine are given to the patient that in a healthy person would cause symptoms of the disease to be relieved.

hypermenorrhea - Also called "menorrhagia," the term refers to excessive blood flow during a woman's period.

insecticide - An agent that kills insects.

infusion - A method of brewing tea in which boiling water is poured over leaves, flowers, or small stems of a plant, and allowed to steep for ten minutes. The process renders a milder tea than a decoction.

laxative - Something that acts gently to promote bowel movements. Purgatives have a stronger effect on the bowels.

liniment - Also called an "embrocation," it is a paste or oily liquid prepared for external application, usually by rubbing into the skin. Liniments alleviate rheumatism, neuralgia, swollen glands, sprains, and bruises.

narcotic - An agent that diminishes the action of the nervous and muscular systems, diminishes pain, induces sleep, stupor, and insensibility.

nervine - Also called a nerve tonic, it is a preparation to calm nervous tension and irritability, and nourish the nervous system. It restores the energy balance within the body.

ointment - Like a liniment, only with a greasier, more solid feel. It is used in the same way as a liniment.

parasiticide - An agent that destroys parasites like tapeworm, lice, liver flukes and bed bugs.

pectoral - Something that eases pain of diseases of the lungs and bronchial tubes.

poultice - A warm, soft, moist plaster applied directly to the skin, then covered with a cloth. The purpose of a poultice is to alleviate inflammations, sores, blood poisoning, bites, and irritated nerve endings. Poultices increase the circulation and ease pain. Do not apply them to open wounds, as they tend to promote bacterial growth.

rubefacient - A substance applied to the skin that increases flow of blood at its surface. It produces redness and may cause the skin to peel from the body where applied. Use rubefacients and other counterirritants in cases of acute and chronic inflammation. They increase circulation.

sedative - A remedy to quiet the central nervous system and induce sleep. If it also soothes pain, it is called an anodyne.

sopoforic - Another remedy to induce sleep.

stimulant - An agent that increases the body's energy reserves, and circulation, breaks up obstructions that have reduced the body's energy, such as prolonged, low-grade fevers, and sluggish digestion. It warms the body by increasing metabolism, and stimulating the system to throw off illness. Not recommended in cases of nervousness, hypertension, ulcerative colitis, or when the body is extremely weak from disease.

stomachic - A tonic that strengthens and tones the stomach, and aids digestion.

syrup - A remedy for a cough or sore throat; an added advantage of a syrup is that it retards the deterioration rates of sensitive herbs. Mix two ounces of the herb required in one part water, boil, strain, and add two ounces honey. A julep is a kind of syrup meant for immediate consumption.

tincture - A concentrated water and alcohol solution, generally of vegetable origin. The final alcohol content is thirty percent or more. To make a tincture, at the new moon, mix four ounces of powdered or cut herb in one pint alcohol. Shake the bottle daily until the full moon. After letting the herbs settle to the bottom, pour off the tincture by straining the liquid through a fine cloth or coffee filter. You may substitute vinegar for alcohol, if you prefer. Administer in doses of one-half to one teaspoonful.

tonic - A tonic promotes the functioning of the body's systems, maintains health, builds energy, and balances. It is ingested as a preventative when no disease is present.

tranquilizer - Something that induces a serene mental state, free from anxiety and agitation.

vermifuge - An agent that kills or expels intestinal worms.

vulnerary - Encourages healing of wounds by promoting cell growth and repair.

II: TEA LEAF SYMBOLS

Perceiving and interpreting images formed by tea leaves is a subjective, intuitive business. The best way to perfect this skill is to keep a notebook of your readings, including the individual meanings of the representations, and how you read them in combination with other signs. Make a diagram of each cup if necessary, showing relative size and positions of the configurations.

Here are some interpretations of figures you are likely to see.

I offer meanings for other symbols in chapter 5.

As you practice, you may evolve other definitions for these symbols which will be valid for you. Remember that any form can hold an actual as well as a symbolic value. For example, although a house means "domestic bliss," it could also refer to an actual house.

Check coupled and other nearby images to refine your interpretations.

ACES

These are all positive signs: hearts - love and happiness; diamonds - a gift, material gain; clubs - a recently initiated project will be successful, a letter; spades - the inquirer will win a battle, a large building.

ACORN

Success; everything will turn out better than hoped for; at the top - financial success; in the middle - better health; at the bottom - both health and financial situation will improve.

ACROBAT

The inquirer is juggling a dicey situation; success after surmounting difficulties.

AIRPLANE

Travel, property, inheritance, promotion; a risky journey or a sudden trip; success after trials and tribulations.

ALLIGATOR

Treachery.

ANCHOR

Success, security, happy results; travel for the good of all concerned; at the top of the cup - success through a lover or through financial endeavors; in the middle of the cup - a successful voyage; at the bottom of the cup - a social occasion will be pleasant and profitable.

ANGEL

The inquirer is protected and providentially provided for; good news.

ANT

Hard work brings gain; thrift.

APPLE

Accomplishment of a goal; gain through education; advice to treat your spouse well, or you may quarrel.

APRON

New friends; the inquirer feels tied close to home.

ARC

An accident or illness.

ARCHWAY

New projects, opportunities; weddings, partnerships; a trip to a faraway destination.

ARROW

News, perhaps not so good.

AX

Troubles are overcome.

BABY

Persistent, small worries; new projects, an actual baby.

BAG

A surprise.

BALL

Restlessness; fortunes bouncing like a ball; sports.

BALLOON

Exaggerated troubles will soon pass.

BASKET

At the top - wealth, bounty; near the handle - a baby;   filled with flowers - social success.

BAT

By tradition, a bat signifies disappointment and a false friend, but I believe it actually signifies protection.

BEANS

Financial distress.

BEAR

Trouble, perhaps because of a delay.

BED

An illness, lack of energy or motivation; time to take a rest.

BEE

Good news, a friend, a busy time; close to handle - a social gathering; a swarm of bees - public success.

BEEHIVE

Prosperity, especially in business.

BEETLE

A difficult task requiring perseverance, but that will turn out well.

BELL

The inquirer will receive or make an announcement; near the top - promotion at work; near the bottom - bad news; bells coupled - joy; many bells - a wedding.

BIRD

Good news, insight, leadership, guidance; if nesting - harmony in the home, love, family; if flying - news to come soon by letter or phone.

BLOTS

If thick and chunky - a warning of a lawsuit; if long and uneven - disappointment.

BOAT

A visitation; refuge from trouble.

BOOK

Higher learning, studious pursuits; more information is needed; advice, lawsuits.

BOOT

Divine protection, achievement; facing away from handle - a dismissal; may refer to Italy.

BOTTLE

A social invitation; conviviality.

BOW

A flirtation, a present.

BOW AND ARROW

A scandal, the zodiac sign Sagittarius.

BOX

Open - romance will prevail; closed - lost property recovered; oblong - the inquirer is hiding something, or someone is hiding something from the inquirer. (Further meanings under SQUARE).

BRACELET

A marriage proposal; a social gathering; a gift.

BRANCH

Bare - disappointment; leafed - a birth.

BRIDGE

An opportunity presents itself; changes; a choice is offered.

BROOM

New beginnings.

BULL

An enemy, quarrels, stubbornness; the zodiac sign Taurus.

BUTTERFLY

Frivolous pursuits, easy pleasures, fickleness; surrounded by dots - frittering away money.

CANDLE

Higher education; thirst for knowledge; help is offered; current situation will improve.

CAGE

A proposal; a loveless marriage.

CAMEL

Useful news; fortitude.

CAP

Trouble, take heed.

CAR

Good luck; a change in surroundings.

CART

Prosperity in business; a delay.

CASTLE

Wish is fulfilled; a strong, successful person; nobility; equity through marriage.

CAT

Psychic development; a link with the occult; striving for independence; a jealous enemy or false friend.

CATTLE

Prosperity.

CAULDRON

Fertility; a birth in the family, or in the mind (the birth of an idea).

CHAIN

An engagement or wedding; unity; constrictions.

CHAIR

Conditions will improve; an unexpected guest; advice to rest.

CHERRIES

A happy love affair.

CHICKEN

Industriousness.

CHILD

An actual child; a promising future, a period of apprenticeship; innocence.

CHURCH

Sudden financial gain, a ceremony; faith, aspirations.

CIGAR

A new friend.

CIRCLE

Completion, good luck; coupled with a dot - pregnancy; cut by lines - disappointment, unfinished business; a delay; if the circle seems like a ring - marriage.

CLOCK

A warning to think of the future and act without delay; a serious illness where immediate action is required; if in the middle of the cup - the patient will recover; at the bottom of the cup - the patient may not recover, or the illness will last a long time; hands of the clock pointing to 7 or 9 - death; hands pointing to 12 - a secret rendezvous for love or profit.

CLOUDS

Trouble.

CLOVER

Prosperity, good luck; inquirer may change lovers.

COAT

Separation, friendship ends.

COCK

Something to crow about; financial independence; do not hesitate.

COLLAR

Dependence.

COMB

Release from small obligations; deceit.

COMPASS

Travel; a change of job; a new direction is required.

CRAB

The zodiac sign Cancer; an enemy.

CRESCENT

Love with an exotic stranger or in a foreign place; a crossroads in life.

CROSS

One - protection; two - a long life; three - a great achievement.

CROWN

A well-earned victory; if very clearly formed - a legacy; honors.

CUP

Reward gained through effort; love, happiness.

DAFFODIL

Wealth, success.

DAGGER

Danger; machinations of enemies; impetuosity.

DASHES

A period of thrills and excitement; advice to follow through on projects.

DESK

A letter brings news concerning business.

DICE

Advice not to gamble now.

DISH

A domestic spat.

DOG

A faithful friend.

DONKEY

Patience, pride.

DOTS

Money, security; a single dot coupled with another symbol emphasizes its meaning.

DRAGON

Challenges, troubles; royalty; a sudden change.

DRUM

A new job; gossip, quarrels.

DUCK

Money, fidelity.

EAGLE

A change for the better; fame attained.

EGG

Prosperity, success; a pregnancy.

ELEPHANT

A trusted friend; wisdom, strength; long-lasting success.

EYE

A caution; someone is watching the inquirer.

FAIRY

A rare sign meaning enchantment, joy, unusually good fortune.

FAN

A flirtation; advice to be discreet.

FEATHER

Energies are scattered; inability to concentrate; instability, inconsistency.

FEET

An important decision.

FENCE

Constriction; success after minor setbacks.

FIR

Success in the arts.

FIRE

Hasty action or reaction, anger; achievement.

FISH

A most fortunate sign; an excellent omen of good fortune and success.

FLAG

Victory; perhaps a warning of danger or quarrels.

FLOWER

Wish fulfilled; success, happiness; bouquet of flowers - joy, prosperity, luck, love.

FORK

Flattery, deceit; a decision that splits feelings.

FROG

Fertility, pregnancy; success comes through changing job or home; egotism.

GARLAND

Honors, success.

GATE

A sudden change in fortune; an opportunity; all is well.

GEESE

Unexpected, but fascinating guests; an invitation.

GLASS

Integrity.

GLOVE

A challenge; justice meted out.

GOAT

News from a sailor; someone is bothering the inquirer; the zodiac sign Capricorn.

GRAPES

Happiness, fulfillment.

GRASSHOPPER

News from a friend away on travels; advice against scattered interests.

GUN

An argument.

HAMMER

Ruthlessness, headaches at work; obstacles will be overcome.

HAND

Friendship; clenched - quarrel.

HARE

Timidity; news from a friend; a crisis needs quick decision and action in order to be averted.

HARP

Harmony, romance, happiness in marriage.

HAT

Someone is hiding something; a new job; change; diplomacy; a rival.

HEART

Love.

HEN

Domestic bliss.

HILL

Obstacles to surmount.

HOE

Hard work leads to success.

HORSE

A lover.

HOUSE

Businesses started now will succeed; domestic harmony.

IRIS

Romance in a garden.

IVY

Friendship; an old house reveals its secrets.

JEWELRY

A gift.

JOCKEY

Speculation; love for a gambler.

JUG

Health, money situation, and reputation improve.

KANGAROO

Domestic harmony.

KEY

Opportunity; doors open; crossed keys - success; double keys - a robbery.

KITE

Wish will be fulfilled; scandal; ambition; dreaming.

KNIFE

Breaking off of relationship abruptly leaving bad feelings.

LADDER

Advancement, probably through hard work.

LAMP

Marriage, a quest; the inquirer's studies may be interrupted by a stranger whom she/he will resent at first, but later will come to appreciate; near rim - a celebration; near handle - money; two lamps - two marriages.

LEAF

Prosperity and good fortune; maple leaf - may refer to Canada, or a Canadian.

LETTERS

Initials of people involved in the inquirer's life; initials that stand for something important in the inquirer's life; written letter - news.

LETTERS

"M" - someone who has the inquirer's best interests at heart; "S" - if reading for a man, he will meet a strikingly beautiful woman; if reading for a woman, with care, she will become more lovely than she ever imagined; "T" - a plan is being hatched; "V" - sex appeal; "X" - crossed paths; "Y" - a choice is offered of two paths to follow.

LINES

Wavy - a warning, uncertainty; parallel - a spiritual journey; straight and clear - progress, trips; slanting downward - business failure; slanting upward - business success.

LION

The zodiac sign Leo; influential friends; ambition, pride.

MASK

Deception, someone is hiding facts from the inquirer.

MERMAID

Temptation, a fascinating sea journey, or fascinating prospects arriving from overseas.

MONKEY

Flattery, mischief; scandal.

MONSTER

Terror.

MOON

Romance, travel, family; full - a love affair; first quarter - new beginnings; last quarter - energy ebbs, fortunes decline, depression.

MUSHROOM

Growth, sometimes uncontrollable; a large obstacle.

MOUSE

A theft; an unassuming person will influence the inquirer's life.

NAIL

An injustice, maliciousness; a sharp pain; an architect.

NECKLACE

Whole - admirers; broken - a relationship ends.

NEEDLE

An admirer; trouble.

NUMBERS

Amounts, dates, etc.; interpret them according to the coupled signs.

NUN

Quarantine; discretion is advised; if reading for a woman, there is a strong desire to leave the cares and woes of the mundane world in order to pursue higher learning and a more spiritual path.

OAK

Strength, long life; the inquirer is favored by the gods.

OAR

Help comes during a difficult situation.

OCTOPUS

Danger.

OLD MAN OR WOMAN

Responsibilities.

OSTRICH

Travel; a warning not to hide from responsibilities.

OVAL

Beware of self-pride.

OWL

Failure; a scandal; wisdom; a night person, or something that will happen at night; a mystery.

OYSTER

Riches; a long courtship; advice to share one's thoughts with others.

PACKAGE

A surprise; a gift.

PAN

Petty anxieties.

PARROT

A trip; scandal, gossip.

PEACOCK

Riches, luxury; property; vanity.

PEAR

Comfort; good fortune.

PENTAGRAM

Protection; balance of mental and physical efforts; white Witchcraft.

PIG

Financial success, but emotional problems, a happy-go-lucky person; a banker.

PIPE

Thoughts; keep an open mind.

PROFILE

A new friend.

PYRAMID

Long-abiding success.

RAIN

Fertilization; depression.

RAVEN

Advice against pessimism.

RIBBONS

Fulfillment. (See BOW)

RIDER

Hasty news.

RIVER

The inquirer's most cherished possession will last forever.

ROCK

Small difficulties.

ROOF

A change in location; a feeling of vulnerability.

ROSE

Happiness, fulfillment; popularity; success in the arts; good children.

SAW

Outside interference.

SCISSORS

A separation.

SEA GULL

Survival; gullibility.

SHELL

Good news; a seaside vacation.

SHOE

A change for the better.

SKELETON

Death, illness, poverty.

SPIDER

Hard work brings success; unexpected money; determination, persistence; intrigue.

SPOON

Generosity.

SQUARE

A tight spot or quandary; suffering, hindrances; protection from accidents.

STAR

Happiness, good luck, health, and fortune.

STEEPLE

A delay.

STICKS

Parallel - change; bent - hesitation; forming a straight line - a happy life; accomplishment, progress; several short, straight sticks - illness; forked - a decision must be made.

SUN

Creativity, happiness, success, growth; honors; a birth.

SWAN

Contentment; mysticism; a lover.

TABLE

A festive gathering; abundance; a business meeting.

TEAPOT

Committee meeting; discussions.

TENT

Travel, vacation.

THIMBLE

Domestic scene changes.

TORCH

Conditions improving; new enthusiastically tackled interests.

TORTOISE

Criticism; difficulties.

TOWER

Either an opportunity or a disaster, depending on how it is aspected.

TREE

Wish fulfillment; changes for the better; endurance, good health.

TRIANGLE

Unexpected news; pointing upward - success; the inquirer is guided by spiritual considerations; pointing downward - failure; a lovers' triangle; the inquirer is ruled by the material plane.

UMBRELLA

Protection; insurance; if closed - trouble.

UNICORN

A secret wedding; chastity; self-sacrifice; problem solved.

VASE

A friend needs help; good deeds; peace of mind.

VIOLET

A walk through the forest will lead to love.

VIOLIN

Individualism, egotism; gaiety.

VULTURE

Although some readers consider it a symbol of loss, theft, and enemies in high places, others believe it to be a symbol of protection.

WAGON

A wedding; a rough future.

WATERFALL

Prosperity.

WHALE

Success in business.

WHEEL

Good fortune, success after hard work; a promotion; near the rim - unexpected money; broken - disappointment.

WINDOW

Open - good luck through a friend; closed - a friend creates disappointment.

WINGS

Messages, usually of a cheerful nature.

III: KINDS OF STONES

QUARTZES

Composition: silicon dioxide.
Stones: agate, amethyst, aventurine, carnelian, cat's eye, chalcedony, chrysoprase, citrine, hawk's eye, heliotrope, jasper, obsidian, onyx, crystal,
rose, quartz, smoky quartz, sardonyx, tiger's eye.

BERYLS

Composition: berylum, aluminum silicate.
Stones: alexandrite, aquamarine, chrysoberyl, emerald, beryls of all types.

CORUNDUMS

Composition: aluminum oxide.
Stones: corundums, jacinth, oriental amethyst, ruby, sapphire, topaz.

FELDSPARS

Composition: aluminum silicate mixed with several other metals; feldspars
are found in igneous rock.
Stones: granite, amazonite, labradorite, moonstone, sunstone.

DIAMONDS

Composition: crystalline carbon.
Stones: diamond, jet, pyrite.

HORNBLENDE

Composition: silicate of calcium and magnesium usually found with zinc,
manganese, and iron.

MICA

A group of complex potassium sodium magnesium, iron aluminum
hydroxyl silicates that crystallize in thin, somewhat flexible, easily separated
layers, which are also translucent or transparent.

OTHER STONES

Animal/Vegetable Kingdoms: amber, coal, coral, pearl, petrified wood (which actually has transformed into silicon dioxide), toadstone.

Pure Volcanic Rock: apache tears (obsidian).

Elements: copper, iron, lead, mercury, silver, sulfur.

Endnotes

1. Sharon Begley and Elizabeth Johnson. "Research Amid the Camellias," *Newsweek* May 15, 1989.

2. Grillot de Givry. *Witchraft, Magic and Alchemy*. p. 187.

3. Charles and Violet Schaefer. *Teacraft*.

4. Catherine of Braganza, Queen to Charles II of England.

5. Isha Mellor. *The Little Tea Book*. p. 7.

6. John Blofeld. *The Chinese Art of Tea*. p. 190.

7. Mitzie Stuart Keller. *Mysterious Herbs and Roots*. p. 377.

8. William Hewitt. *Tea Leaf Reading*. p. 1.

9. Faber Birren. *Color Psychology and Color Therapy*. p. 197.

10. Jonathan Gash. *Pearlhanger*. pp. 112-13.

11. Anna Riva. *The Modern Herbal Spellbook*. p. 5.

12. Aima. *Ritual Book of Herbal Spells*. p.40.

13. M. Grieve. *A Modern Herbal*. vol. I. p. 249.

14. *A Modern Herbal*. vol I. p. 290.

15. Sarah Morrison. *The Modern Witch's Spellbook*. vol II. pp. 27-28.

16. Miguel Tierra. *The Way of Herbs*. p. 101.

17. *The Modern Witches Spellbook*. vol. II. p. 77.

18. Aima. *Ritual Book of Herbal Spells*. p. 114.

Bibliography

Aima. *Ritual Book of Herbal Spells.* New, Enlarged, Revised Edition. U.S.A.: Foibles Publications, 1980 rpt 1976.

Anon. *The Ancient Book of Formulas.* Dallas: Dorene Publishing Co., Inc., 1967.

Beyerl, Paul. *The Master Book of Herbalism.* Custer, Washington: Phoenix Publishing Co., 1984.

Birren, Faber. *Color Psychology and Color Therapy: A Factual Study of the Influence of Color in Human Life.* Secaucus, New Jersey: The Citadel Press, 1961 rpt 1950.

Blofeld, John. *The Chinese Art of Tea.* Boston: Shambhala Publications, Inc., 1985.

Carter, Lady Sara. *The Book of Light.* Magickal Childe Publishing, Inc., 1974.

Cavendish, Richard. *The Black Arts.* New York: G.P. Putnam's Sons, 1967.

Chamberlain, Mary. *Old Wives' Tales.* London: Virago Press, 1981.

Cirlot, J. E. *A Dictionary of Symbols.* 2nd. Ed. Translated by Jack Sage. New York: Philosophical Library, 1983 rpt 1962.

Conway, David *Ritual Magic: An Occult Primer.* New York: E.P. Dutton, 1978 rpt 1972.

Cooper, J. C. *Symbolism: The Universal Language.* Great Britain: The Aquarian Press, 1982.

Crow, W. B., *The Occult Properties of Herbs and Plants.* New York: Samuel Weiser Inc., 1976 rpt 1969.

------ *Precious Stones: Their Occult Power and Hidden Significance.* Great Britain: The Aquarian Press, 1980 rpt 1968.

Crowther, Patricia. *Lid Off the Cauldron: A Handbook for Witches.* London: Frederick Muller Ltd., 1981.

Culpeper, Nicholas. *Culpeper's Complete Herbal.* London: W. Faulsham and Co., Ltd., nd.

De Givry, Grillot *Witchcraft, Magic and Alchemy.* Translated by J. Courteny Locke. New York: Dover Publications, Inc., 1985.

Editors "The Witch's Garden" in *Witches and Witchcraft, Mysteries of the Unknown Series.* Alexandria, Virginia: Time-Life Books, 1990.

Evelyn, Nancy. *The Herbal Medicine Chest.* Freedom, California: The Crossing Press, 1989.

Fontana, Marjorie A. *Cup of Fortune: A Guide to Tea Leaf Reading.* Madison, Wisconsin: Fontastic, 1979.

Gamache, Henri. *The Magic of Herbs.* Highland Falls, New York: Sheldon Publications, 1942.

Grieve, M. *A Modern Herbal,* vols. I and II. New York: Dover Publications, Inc., 1971 rpt 1931.

Hewitt, William. *Tea Leaf Reading.* St. Paul: Llewellyn Publications, Inc., 1989.

Junius, Manfred M. *Practical Handbook of Plant Alchemy: How to Prepare Medicinal Essences, Tinctures and Elixirs.* Translated by Leóne Muller. New York: Inner Traditions International, Ltd., 1985.

Kamm, Minnie Watson. *Old-Time Herbs for Northern Gardens.* New York: Dover, 1971 rpt 1938.

Keller, Mitzie Stuart. *Mysterious Herbs and Roots: Ancient Secrets for Beautie, Health, Magick, Prevention and Youth.* Culver City, California: Peace Press, Inc., 1978.

Kordel, Lelord. *Natural Folk Remedies.* New York: G. P. Putnam's Sons, 1974.

Mathers, S. L. MacGregor. *The Greater Key of Solomon.* Chicago: De Laurence Scott and Co., 1914.

------*The Grimoire of Armadel.* York Beach, Maine: Samuel Weiser, Inc., 1983 rpt 1980.

------ *The Lesser Key of Solomon.* Edited by L.L. de Laurence. Chicago: De Laurence Scott, 1916.

McCleod, Dawn. *Herb Handbook: A Practical Guide to Herbs and Their Uses.* North Hollywood: Wilshire Book Co., 1968.

McWharter, Margaret Lange. *Tea Cup Tales: Tales of Tea and How to Read Tea Leaves.* Ramona, California: Ransom Hill Press, 1984.

Medsger, Oliver Perry. *Edible Wild Plants.* New York: Collier Books, 1966 rpt 1939.

Mellor, Isha. *The Little Tea Book.* Great Britain: Judy Piathus Publishers, Ltd., 1985.

Moore, Michael. *Medicinal Plants of the Mountain West.* Santa Fe: The Museum of New Mexico Press, 1988 rpt 1980.

Morrison, Sarah Lyddon. *The Modern Witch's Spellbook.* Book II. Secaucus, New Jersey: Citadel Press, 1986.

Neto, Texeira. *Pomba-Gira: Rituals to Invoke the Formidable Powers of the Female Messenger of the Gods.* Translated by Carol L. Dow. Burbank, California: Technicians of the Sacred, 1992.

Petalengro, Gipsy. *Romany Herbal Remedies.* North Hollywood: Newcastle Publishing Co., Inc., 1982.

Poinsot, M. C. *The Encyclopedia of Occult Sciences.* New York: Tudor Publishing Company, 1968 rpt 1939.

Readers' Digest Association, Inc. *Magic and Medicine of Plants.* New York: The Readers Digest Association, Inc., 1986.

Regardie, Israel *How to Make and Use Talismans.* New York: Samuel Weiser, Inc., 1972.

------*The Art of True Healing.* Great Britain: Servants of the Light Association, 1977 rpt 1937.

Ricli, Franco Maria. *Herbarium.* Translated by Michael Langley. New York: Rizzoli International Publications, Inc., 1980.

Riva, Anna. *The Modern Herbal Spellbook: The Magical Uses of Herbs.* Toluca Lake, California: International Imports, 1974.

------ *The Modern Witchcraft Spellbook.* Toluca Lake, California: International Imports, 1972.

Rohde, Eleanour Sinclair. *A Garden of Herbs.* Revised and Enlarged Edition. New York: Dover, 1969 rpt 1936.

Rose, Jeanne. *Herbs and Things.* New York: Grossett and Dunlap, 1972.

Schaefer, Charles and Violet. *Teacraft.* San Francisco: Yerba Buena Press, 1975.

Schoen, Linda Allen, ed. *The AMA Book of Skin and Hair Care.* Philadelphia and New York: J. B. Lippincott Co., 1976 rpt 1971.

Thomas, William, and Pavitt, Kati. *The Book of Talismans, Amulets and Zodiacal Gems.* North Hollywood: Wilshire Book Co, 1970 rpt 1914

Tierra, Michael. *The Way of Herbs.* Santa Cruz, California: Unity Press, 1989.

Uyldert, Mellie. *The Psychic Garden: Plants and Their Esoteric Relationship with Man.* Translated by H.A. Smith. Great Britain: Thorsons Publishers Ltd., 1980

Walker, Barbara G. *The Book of Sacred Stones: Fact and Fallacy in the Crystal World.* San Francisco: Harper and Row Publishers, 1989.

Wright, Elbee. *Book of Legendary Spells: A Collection of Unusual Legends from Various Ages and Cultures.* Minneapolis: Marlar Publishing Co., 1974 rpt 1968.